GOING
WITH
MY GUT

*How Intuition Healed
My Body—and My Life*

CARRIE ECKERT

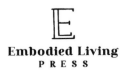

Embodied Living
P R E S S

Published and distributed by Embodied Living Press in Sarasota, FL
www.embodiedlivingpress.com

Library of Congress Control Number: 2021905366

ISBN 978-1-7364742-0-4 (paperback)
ISBN 978-1-7364742-1-1 (EPUB)

Editors: Ellen Brown and Allison Serrell
Cover and interior design: Morgan Krehbiel
Author photograph: Daniel Perales

Produced by Wonderwell
www.wonderwell.press

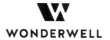

Printed and bound in the US

For Matt

These rough waters of life are constantly made
smoother by your unfailing love and commitment.
You've always encouraged me to go with my gut.
For that I am so very grateful.

CONTENTS

NOTE TO READER

This story is based on my life and experiences as I remember them. A few names and characteristics have been changed in the interest of privacy.

INTRODUCTION

IN 2012, I CONTRACTED A RESPIRATORY VIRUS from which I only partially recovered. The illness I suffered from had no explanation, no prognosis, and the absence of an explanation stripped my suffering of its legitimacy. To be ill with no known cause was to live as an outsider. Even within my own body.

Like countless other women and men with undiagnosed illnesses, I consulted medical practitioners who dismissed my symptoms as being my own mind's creation, part of the package of becoming a new mom, or the result of untreated depression. The inability of Western medicine to diagnose my illness meant the illness did not exist.

My experience in and through "dis-ease" followed a circuitous route over a period of many years going as far back as my early twenties. I use the hyphenated form of the word disease because ease, by definition, means comfort of body or mind (and freedom from pain or trouble) and dis comes from the Latin prefix meaning apart; so dis-ease is an unnatural interruption of or a departure from ease. The virus I contracted in 2012 was the tipping point in my health. My overburdened body grew increasingly weary, and I began to suffer ailments ranging from punishing fatigue and headaches to constant brain fog, ever-changing pains throughout my body, and extreme digestive distress.

Like many, I endured despite the frustration and the loneliness until I eventually learned that my body was fully equipped to heal herself. I just needed to listen to her wisdom—to turn inward, to pay attention, to just be. That is how I found the path to wellness.

This book is the story of that journey. I am sharing it with you in the hopes that it may serve as a guide, accompany you in your own search for health and wellness, and help you find your way back to the ease that is your natural birthright.

CHAPTER 1

Leopardess

MANY PEOPLE HAVE TOLD ME THAT I AM AN OLD soul. For most of my life, I have been a bit of a loner among my peers. I began to realize as a preteen that I wasn't going to find my identity in a clique. When friendships became more about social status and false facades than the collaborative and carefree exploration of life, I began to retreat. In high school, the popular crowd didn't seem to notice me, and I felt invisible in their presence. Where I approached the world modestly and reeking of self-doubt, they cocooned themselves inside their fabric of external beauty and confidence. I couldn't possibly have entered their tight circle. Then again, maybe I didn't really want to. Life felt lonely at times, but I got used to it. So when my first adult friendship ended before it had truly begun, I was hurt but not surprised.

In 2000 my husband Matt was serving his four-year tour of duty in the army at Fort Stewart in Hinesville, Georgia. We chose to live in nearby Savannah, a charming antebellum city known for its rich history and haunting yet seductive Spanish moss, where we had fun exploring famous restaurants and reveling at the nation's second-largest yearly St. Patrick's Day parade. As we settled into our new home, I met the wives and girlfriends of the other lieutenants in the army world and found these women to be refreshingly different from the girl packs of my past. They were certainly more mature and accepting. Most of them were building a life around the military; however, I felt a strong pull to make my mark in the business world, where I was working as a sales rep for a pharmaceutical company. Because of this difference in family dynamics, I once again began to feel like an outsider—until I met Christy. Christy was a real estate agent who managed the apartment complex where I lived. Like me, she was independent and took her husband's deployments and late nights in stride. She was just as dedicated to her career as she was supportive of her husband's commitment to serving his country. She was gregarious, outspoken, and ambitious, and I felt at ease with her in a way that I had not with so many other women. She was a no-nonsense friend who could always be counted on to dispense the hard truth.

One day a few months after Christy and I met, my company's most important account, a physician's office, ran low on samples of the premier drug we supplied them. If we could not restock these, the doctor would likely replace us with another player in the industry. Other than marketing materials and Big Pharma-funded studies, not much differentiated one drug from another in those days, so sales success depended on schmoozing and customer service. My sales partner (who stood to earn us a lavish trip to Paris as a reward for keeping the doctor's business) needed me to step in and cover this account for her that day.

A shipment of these medication samples was scheduled to arrive at my apartment by early afternoon. I rushed home after my lunch appointment to be there as soon as my friendly FedEx driver arrived. I had filled my trunk with company-branded tchotchkes and homemade brownies, perfectly wrapped with color-coordinated bows, ready to give away with the all-important medication samples. With my garage wide open and trunk ajar, I stood there waiting.

It was another gorgeous sun-drenched winter day in Georgia. Herons waded among the surrounding marsh grasses; a flock of black skimmers made a fluid formation against a backdrop of fluffy clouds. At least that is how I imagine the day was, but my attention was solely focused on the arms of my watch as they made their way around the dial. Minutes passing, my anger grew as this completely irresponsible, slacker of a FedEx driver was taking her sweet time.

Why the hell was she allowed to work for such an esteemed company, one well-known for its dedication to assuring that parcels were delivered to recipients throughout the world promptly, I asked myself. *She won't last long in this business. As soon as those boxes arrive, I am going to get in touch with her boss and rip her a new one! This will be her very last delivery if I have anything to say about it.*

You can imagine the shitstorm that ensued when she showed up. (If you do not have your own inner leopardess this might be more difficult to understand. It makes little logical sense. After all, we are talking about a box of acid reflux pills, not a life-or-death situation.)

"You're *two* hours late!" I screamed at her in a voice that demanded the entire planet and every person on it should have revolved around me and my schedule. "What the hell were you doing? I literally have five minutes to drive all the way across town to get these samples to my most important account, or I'll lose my freakin' job," I ranted, exaggerating a bit. "Do you really think I'm going to be able to make it at this point? And what about all the appointments I canceled to do this one *very critical thing* today?" Knowing it was too late to get there, I yanked the packages out of her hand and threw them into a scattered mess in the garage.

She froze, eyes wide, and then sheepishly apologized before climbing back into her truck and driving away. With no time left to make it to my important account, everything suddenly got quiet. Too quiet. I stood there, reticent, unwilling to face the embarrassment of what had just unfolded. Instead, I remained indignant and called my partner with the bad news. I had failed my mission. And it was all the FedEx lady's fault.

Amid the afternoon frenzy, my inner leopardess had been summoned, and when my leopardess is in charge, she knows she has to stand her ground to survive. Like the leopardess who lives under threat of extinction, my instincts at that moment were to protect my job, and therefore my identity, at all costs.

I wish I could say the story ended there. The FedEx driver had stopped by the apartment complex office to apologize to, yep, Christy. Unable to explain to me the reason for her delay as she stood frozen in fear of my wrath, she wanted to let the rest of the residents know they could count on her to make their deliveries in a timely manner. Later, Christy called my husband to express concern about my mental state. As it turned out, the FedEx driver I ripped up one side and down the other had been handling someone else's crisis that day. The local hospital found themselves in need of an emergency transplant, and she was tasked with transporting a human organ from one end of town to the other before a 52-year-old man died on the operating table. And for her efforts to save a man's life, she got to meet me and my leopardess.

Unfortunately, my behavior outside the apartment garage that day was a pivotal moment in my relationship with Christy—one that just wasn't salvageable. I felt that my public display of anger had terrified her, and afterwards she looked at me with a hint of fear in her eyes, as if she expected her friend might morph into a crazed lunatic. My angry outbursts had been known to come out of nowhere and alienate family and friends at times growing up, but I never felt as though I had truly lost anyone close to me because of them (until now).

My inner leopardess was adept at protecting me for a large portion of my life. The rage I felt in my early twenties was the continuation of a pattern that had taken root in me at a very early age. Understanding the structure of this root and getting to know its parts—parts with names like unworthiness and shame—eventually became an integral role in my healing.

I have learned that anger is the greatest defender of my sadness, and all the health-promoting diets, medicines, and holistic protocols could only take me so far until I was willing to lower my shield and connect my ailing body with my mind. That was when the real healing occurred, and I truly began living again.

CHAPTER 2

Symptoms

LESS THAN A YEAR LATER, MY HUSBAND COMPLETED his commitment to the army, and we moved to the small town of Macon, Georgia. His time in the service allowed us to buy a picturesque Victorian house with a VA loan close to a few eclectic downtown restaurants and wine tasting venues. We enjoyed three relatively carefree years in our oddly endearing southern town.

While we both excelled in our sales careers, I found myself a frequent patient in the same doctors' offices in which I sold medications. Anyone who has had constant sinus allergies can understand how inelegant the condition. A steady stream of mucus had dripped from my nose since childhood, necessitating regular doctor visits and the ever-present wad of tissues in my backpack, my purse, and now my pharmaceutical sales bag. Told by numerous doctors that the grasses and trees in my home state of North Carolina had triggered me, I had been lethargic with a cloudy head of sinus congestion for as long as

I could remember. Apparently, the flora in Georgia was having the same effect.

I was sensitive to several different pollens, a few molds, dust mites, cat and dog dander, and cockroaches, my new allergist reported. "Have you noticed that these bother you?" he asked gently.

It sounded about right, but . . . dogs? *I'm not allergic to Maddie!* I thought, feeling disheartened. An image of our springer spaniel's sweet expectant face greeting me through the front door glass when I came home at the end of a long workday came to mind.

He suggested allergen immunotherapy injections as he extended a hand to help me down from the exam table. I had been managing my nasal problems with medication for as long as I could remember. Doctors rotated me through every corticosteroid on the market attempting to land on one that would eliminate the nasal drip that left my nose raw. Nothing worked completely or without side effects. I took these prescriptions to manage the congestion but still coated my nostrils with Vaseline to deal with the nose-bleeds the medicine induced. I also kept albuterol around for the occasional wheezing I had on particularly bad days.

If I wanted to be seen by my customers as a dedicated colleague and not just another day patient, I figured I had no choice but to go with the gold standard of allergy treat-ment: weekly immunotherapy shots. But something I did not yet understand was keeping me from moving forward. "Are allergy shots safe?" I asked, not sure how to be more specific. Injecting a small dose of pollen or dust under my skin did not seem harmful; we are exposed to those irritants in the air all the time. Yet my gut was telling me something did not make sense.

Allergen immunotherapy is more than one hundred years old and has few side effects, he assured me. They even monitored patients for thirty minutes after the shot to be cautious. This did not address my true concern, which was more about negative long-term effects than acute reactions. I was more hung up on things like going blind, becoming paralyzed, having my tongue fall out—things that couldn't be undone. Had anyone studied long-term effects on patients? I was too reluctant to ask this and too concerned about straining the conversation and sounding like I was questioning his authority.

"How long will I need to get the shots?" I asked instead, dreading the idea of spending hours driving across town every week.

"It could take up to three years to desensitize your immune system," he said. "The goal is to allow it to build up a tolerance to the pollen and dust that trigger a reaction in you, ideally reducing or eliminating the symptoms. This is a gradual process."

"I'll think about it and let you know," I replied as I picked up my leather bag to dig around for a tissue. Feeling defeated, I asked for a refill of my Veramyst nasal spray, which he was happy to provide.

Something just did not feel right, but I had not yet acknowledged the subtle signals from my body as instructions instead of inconvenient physical sensations to be ignored. At the time I did not know anything about adjuvants like aluminum and phenol that are commonly used as preservatives in allergy shots. I did not yet know that my body might be too fragile to handle the additional burden of heavy metals and environmental toxins that, in this case, would be injected into me on a regular basis. I just felt reluctant to take this path, which seemed extreme. That sudden tightening in my stomach was strong enough to give me pause. I resigned myself to managing my dripping nose as I had all my life by toting around snot rags and snorting steroids.

In addition to my clogged sinuses, another symptom showed annually in the lab work from my wellness checkup. I had low white and red blood cell counts, which seemed (at least to me) to correlate with my uncanny ability to catch a head or chest cold every other month. My doctors seemed to dismiss any concerns I had about a weak immune system, never gave me recommendations for preventing the colds, and suggested I take multivitamins and iron supplements to manage my low blood cell counts.

These simple solutions left me with the message that I must be fine because my doctors simply prescribed the remedies I requested to manage the allergies and never suggested follow-up appointments. I tried to assure myself that I was okay because my medical team indicated that my blood work was only slightly out of range and I looked healthy on the outside.

But I was not convinced, and I continued to feel like the real me was invisible to my doctors. *Maybe I am just a hypochondriac,* I thought. Did doctors think these were trivial problems and that I was wasting their time and taking resources away from their more critical patients?

I certainly did not want to distract them from helping people who needed their care, but I knew something was not right. I wanted to know what was wrong with me, or at the very least, I wanted to feel more robust.

Although I was not aware for many more years that it was atypical, I had also been challenged by constipation my entire life. I can remember sheepishly reaching for the fiber-filled, bowel-enhancing Raisin Bran as everyone else grabbed their candy bars during various summer camps and enrichment programs.

Daily management of my sluggish digestion became second nature to me growing up. But here I was, a decade later and in my twenties, creating gridlock in an already bottlenecked colon with iron supplements meant to treat the low blood count. The blockage-causing mineral that was meant to support my red blood cells exacerbated my constipation which then had to be further offset with Metamucil, glycerin suppositories, and various laxatives. Such was life, I told myself, trying not to recognize any nagging concern.

Most of my early marriage in my twenties were happy-go-lucky years as I simply patched up my little sinus, constipation, and blood count issues and moved on. I even made it through my first pregnancy without so much as a strange food aversion or hormonal rage incident. However, a fourth symptom began to emerge during my first pregnancy as I began to experience fatigue unlike anything my typically energetic body and mind ever had before. Normal when carrying a new life inside you? Definitely. But when I traveled to visit a friend in the middle of my pregnancy in 2003 to help her prepare for her own baby's upcoming birth and found myself the one laid up on the couch most of the day, I was a bit baffled. The second trimester was supposed to be the easiest, but I just was not able to push through the weariness that weekend. Standard baby-creating bodily response? Maybe. Or perhaps this budding fatigue was my newest physical warning sign, a harbinger of the struggles to come.

Overall, both of my pregnancies and the early days with my infants were probably fairly normal, though it never feels that way to an exhausted new mother. The choice to quit my job and stay at home after my first son was born in January 2004 quickly led to feelings of isolation. My lack of creative and intellectual outlets prompted a growing resentment of my husband's freedom to mingle with society via his job. By the time he got home from work, I was ready to throw a slobbery rubber dump truck at his head and came dangerously close a few times! Physically, he survived those years unscathed, but he certainly suffered my angry verbal wrath on more than one occasion.

"How's my little Frodo today?" Matt would ask affectionately as soon as he walked in the door and put down his keys. Frodo was the nickname we had officially bestowed upon Colin when he came out of my womb small and skinny with feet as large as a toddler's.

"I think he looks kind of like a Hobbit," he had proclaimed jokingly, knowing full well that he was the most beautiful baby ever to grace this world.

"You take him. I'm done!" I would bark as I shoved Colin into his waiting arms. When I had reached mental exhaustion, I would march upstairs to rest with the expectation that he would take over exactly where I had left off while I took a much-needed respite. But I typically came back down, unable to resist the urge to micromanage the diaper changes, feedings, and baths, never done my way— the *correct* way.

Throughout my life, when my world got turned upside down, I grasped for a sense of control to feel more stable. Now that the responsibility of protecting and raising a little human had become my overwhelming reality, I sought comfort in trying to perfect every aspect of my immediate surroundings. The sleep deprivation that came along with being a new mom not only left my body weary, but I also struggled with mental energy and clarity. Peace of mind could only be experienced, I felt, if all child-rearing duties were done the way I deemed fit no matter how senseless. Yes, the two dozen stuffed animals needed to be placed back in their proper nooks and the diapers needed to be neatly stacked on the changing table shelf every day, thank you very much.

Compounding my ever-increasing need to control my environment, our son, like many newborns, was not interested in sleeping much at night like the rest of the world. When all the soothing tricks in all the baby books failed, I started climbing into the crib with him until he (and I) finally fell back asleep.

Thankfully at nine months old Colin started sleeping through the night, but before I was able to appreciate this relatively normal milestone, my anxiety set in. Now that extreme exhaustion was no longer knocking me out as soon as he went down, my mind and body were alive enough to create and respond to all manner of irrational fears. Would he die of sudden infant death syndrome (SIDS) because I allowed him to sleep on his stomach? Would his little infant self see me at my worst slamming the breast pump across the room when I could not stand feeling like a cow with worn udders anymore? Would my competence as a mother determine the fate of his future?

Ironically enough, unending exhaustion had transformed into an inability to sleep and I could now only nod off for a few hours at a time. My heart raced and mind swirled as Matt snored blissfully beside me. The only relief from the anarchy taking place in my mind came when I went to check on my son to be sure he was still alive. I often ended up on the floor beside his crib, nodding off as his gentle hums of breath lulled me back to sleep.

Habits began to form during that period of intense insomnia that would take many years to break. Every time I checked the clock, I counted how much time was left before the next day was to begin. How far had I slipped from achieving those needed eight hours of sleep? The more I obsessed about the clock and my required shuteye, the less able I was to actually shut my eyes. Mixing my desire for control with my growing fear of fatigue left me staring at the ceiling and pacing the hallways at night. I inevitably felt as though I had been pummeled by a real dump truck in the morning.

I dragged myself and my fatigued body through the days, feeling only a dull sense of joy when Colin shared a sweet little smile or reached his next baby milestone.

Fortunately, the insomnia resolved over some time with the help of books I read on tamping down anxiety and crippling thoughts. I didn't know then that some of these same Jedi mind tricks would be revisited and modified for new health challenges down the road. This period of insomnia had lasted six very long months and had created yet another fear which would plague me for years to come—the fear of being tired.

◎ ◎ ◎

In 2005 my husband's company transferred us to Jacksonville, Florida. We spent the next decade in a coastal suburb of this larger Florida city, and for many of those years I felt relatively healthy. Colin's childhood and the arrival of our second son, Bennett, brought our family all the love, adventure, and challenges of any happy household. My creative inclinations were satisfied by starting an at-home stationery design business. I found a lot of fulfillment designing wedding invitations and holiday photo cards for clients around the country. This creative endeavor, though, eventually became problematic as my perfectionism—another result of my need to control—crept in.

Planning and preparing the boys' birthday parties, which was one of my greatest joys, turned into a kind of mania, too. As a graphic designer, I loved showcasing my creativity in the form of elaborately themed invitations, color-matched goodie bags, and party decor. As much as I enjoyed expressing myself through design, however, somewhere along the way I crossed the line between creative expression and neurosis. Over time, these parties became more about me and my persona than about the kids and their fun. Thankfully, Colin and Bennett were still too young to know how much the preparation consumed me.

During the manic planning for Colin's fifth birthday celebration, I had been ignoring persistent wheezing and general malaise. On the big day, I ended up in the ER instead of joining a dozen little boys making chocolate covered strawberries and caramel apples. I battled a raspy cough and the pneumonia I was diagnosed with during my visit to the hospital for the next two months and eventually received a vaccine usually given to the high-risk elderly. Everybody else was fine.

The perfectionism that probably contributed to my health challenges may have also awoken my sleeping leopardess. While perfecting my world brought a temporary sense of calm to a chaotic mind, when those controlling efforts failed to deliver on their perceived promise, unleashing my inner leopardess became the next step in my lifelong coping process.

For example, my patience was put to the test every time we prepared to pack up the family and head out on the road for vacation. The tension would start brewing a few days before, and Matt could sense the impending battle as soon as the elaborate checklists, color-coordinated outfit piles, and detailed dog care instructions (scheduled to the minute) appeared on notes throughout the house.

In the summer of 2011 we were preparing for a trip to the Carolinas for a much-needed break from the sweltering Florida heat.

"Is that bag ready for me to take to the car?" Matt asked, his hand hovering over the handle of my suitcase.

"No. The bag will be ready when I'm ready. You know that! I tell you that every freakin' time we go somewhere. Why do you continue to rush me like this?" I yelled from the bathroom as I threw mini bottles of toiletries into my cosmetic bag.

"I was just askin'," he replied in his goofy playful voice. It would take me years to realize this was not his way of mocking me but more his method of shrugging off my volatile energy. It was as if I wanted a target for my mounting stress-turned-anger.

"Well stop ask-ING," I corrected, stomping into the family room where the boys sat glued to the TV. "And maybe do something productive like make sure the boys have both emptied their bladders and put on their shoes so that when I'm packed, we'll be ready to go. Dammit, Matt, why do I have to do everything?" I screamed. It was ironic, really, since the whole conflict had started with his offer to help.

As I stood there, my favorite pillow folded in half under one arm, a huge plastic bag full of goldfish and squeezable applesauce packets hooked on the other arm, and a stack of laundry wedged between my open palms and chin, I noticed four-year-old Bennett's big blue eyes staring up at me with what appeared to my misguided mind to be compassion. I took a deep breath, and we eventually made it out the door and onto the road. My mood shifted and I nodded off to sleep as we pulled onto the freeway, leaving Matt and the kids to absorb the tension I had created.

Keeping my anger in check was not an issue once I was in vacation mode, but a chance meeting with an insidious toxin at the end of the trip opened my mind to a trigger that I would later learn had a sneaky way of exacerbating that temper of mine. After a lovely visit with my mother in the North Carolina mountains, we rounded out our summer adventures with a stop in Charleston, South Carolina. This ended up including an impromptu visit with my college roommate, Beth, who was renting a beach house near our hotel. We spent the day on the beach together, lazily swinging on the hammocks and playing monster tag with Beth's husband and their two little boys.

After the sun finally set behind us and the lively squawks of the seagulls quieted, we corralled everyone inside to prepare for dinner. As I helped Beth peel the skin off the oranges that would tide the kids over until our spaghetti and meatballs would be ready, I was captivated by how effortlessly our boys were getting along. Not knowing when we would visit again, I decided that staying overnight there was a way to keep this magic alive a little longer.

The house was old and musty, but it reminded me of summers at our family's 1940s beach house on the North Carolina coast. That night my heartbeat was unable to settle enough to give my body the calm it needed to drift off to sleep, but I assumed it was just too hot in the room or the dust from the old curtains bothered me. The next morning, my eyes were puffy and I felt both jittery and sluggish, kind of like a bad hangover, though I had only had one glass of wine the night before. I must have been allergic to something, I thought. Feeling not quite right, I made the tough decision to decline an invitation to stay over a second night. As disappointing as it was to the kids and adults alike, we hung around for a few hours and then made our way back to the hotel in town for a restful night before traveling home to Florida.

The beach house seemed to be an isolated allergy incident, and I thought little of it until that fall when we went to Blowing Rock, North Carolina, for my grandmother's ninetieth birthday weekend. The first morning after we had arrived I awoke with a throbbing headache and a face so haggard no amount of makeup could hide my lack of sleep. Once again, I had spent the night staring at the ceiling as my racing heart kept me from capturing more than spurts of sleep. With some twenty or so children and grandchildren gathered to celebrate on this unusually warm November weekend in the heart of the Blue Ridge mountains, there was not room for all of us in one house. The neighbors had graciously offered theirs, and Matt and I were given a bedroom in their furnished basement— their moldy, furnished basement. We could not see visible black spots on the walls or fuzzy green fungal growth in the bathroom crevices, but that familiar mustiness was an obvious warning sign. When my aunt offered me an Ambien to help me sleep the next night, I gladly accepted the little pink pill.

After that weekend in North Carolina, my energy rapidly declined. Whether it was falling asleep while waiting in carpool line to pick up the kids or looking around for the nearest chair within minutes of joining friends, I constantly felt exhausted. But as a mom of two young boys, I wrote off my waning energy as just another adventure in parenting.

I did recognize at this point that I wanted more meaningful relationships. In retrospect, could that have had something to do with my growing weariness? Was I lonely? Though I had two kids, part time design work, and a house to run, I often found myself yearning for that rare type of connection I had had with Christy during our military days in Savannah. I was not able to recreate that bond with the moms at the playground or the women at the gym with our friendly but shallow conversations. Each of those interactions seemed like we were merely treading on the surface of a deep pool, and I longed to dive into those stories of heartbreak and wonder, awe and regret. I began to realize that as much as I had avoided the company of women in the past, now that this companionship was being denied me altogether, I craved meaningful relationships with female friends.

CHAPTER 3
Growing Up

LOOKING BACK, I CAN TRACE MY VOLATILE DIGES-
tion, my anger, and my desire to be seen and heard to an
early age. (Could they all be linked?) A medley of childhood
issues over the years created an inner emotional environment that manifested in my intense need for control.

The first of these was born of my bowel troubles. I was
a colicky baby. Fed on formula, which was in vogue at the
time, my mother spent much of that first year of my life
trying to find a recipe that I would peacefully consume.
She eventually settled on goat's milk. The colic finally
under control, I encountered a particularly troublesome
run-in with dysentery after a family vacation in Europe
when I was two. Not knowing exactly what they were
dealing with, the military doctors in Germany instructed
my parents to feed me a liquids-only diet. No solid foods
were allowed until I produced a firm stool. I drank only
liquids for days until everything I excreted was clear. Solid
stools beyond little pellets never appeared, so my obedient

mother took me back to the hospital to find herself being chastised by another doctor. He said they were starvation stools! She drove me back to our temporary German home and proceeded to shovel food into my weak starving body. She was a new mother in a foreign country. She had taken the man in the white lab coat literally.

Whatever the root cause, the dysentery event was not an isolated gastrointestinal incident. A year and a half later, I complained of tummy aches to my mother and apparently had not pooped in more than two weeks. She took me to the doctor, who examined my abdomen and instructed my parents to go home and give me four to five adult enemas—stat—to dislodge the obstruction. When the fluid contained in four of these plastic squirt bottles failed to get my bowels moving, my parents went for the fifth. I remember lying on the bed, the crisp sheets muffling my screams, as a cold probe was forced into my backside. Fortunately, the fifth enema did its job, and I made it to my best friend's birthday party before the cake arrived to grab a paper hat and stuff my face with gloriously sweet piped icing.

The second issue stemmed from growing up in a military family. Navy life required that we move around a lot during the first five years of my life. My father spent few special occasions with us as he traveled most of the time, and I didn't see him very much. I can only guess that my little self both loved those rare moments together and felt protective of my easily broken heart. How can anyone, especially a child with no understanding of time's great depths, give her heart entirely to someone who leaves for

nine months at a time? What stories could I have con-
cocted to make sense of this person leaving? Was I to
blame? Was I fearful or anxious upon his return, maybe
even unable to remember him?

Perhaps this second issue, the internal emotional strife
I felt during those years, had something to do with the first,
my sluggish digestion. Chronic constipation was something
I had lived with and mostly dismissed my entire life. I did
not know what normal elimination schedules looked like,
as this wasn't something openly discussed in our household.
I imagine my digestive tract also took a bit of a hit in light of
all the bleach I consumed in the water in Iran—the purifi-
cation strategy of choice to protect ourselves from a lack of
sanitation methods.

These issues were also both entwined with a third:
wanting to be the good girl. In elementary school, I became
an expert at holding back—or so I thought. One day in
the third grade, my little eight-year-old mind was in over-
drive as I stood, blinded by stage lights, above a sea of my
peers out ahead as part of the school's much-anticipated
math bee. A numbers parade marched across my brain
each time someone else was asked a question and I would
silently compute the equation myself. Suddenly I realized
I had a more pressing issue. I needed to pee. Badly.

The girl beside me raised her hand.

"May I go to the bathroom?" she asked politely.

Did she just hear my thoughts? Did I say that out loud? I
worried, struggling not to wiggle or call attention to myself.
But then the boy two kids down from me spoke up.

"I need to go, too," he announced.

What? But I need to go! And now I'm really stuck. Every-one will think I'm making it up, I thought, as I contracted my bladder muscles with all the force I could muster.

I continued to play the part of the good girl and stayed in my place on the stage. I was up next. There was absolutely no way I could have interrupted the competition to go to the bathroom at that point.

Uh oh, what's that warm sensation moving down my leg? I thought in horror. Then I noticed my shorts beginning to billow out as if my underwear was a balloon filling with water. I looked out at the audience and smack dab into the eyes of the little boy I was in love with (unbeknownst to him). I was escorted off stage, red face hanging low, muttering apologies.

The fourth underlying thread of my childhood came from my parents' divorce. When they split in 1984, my mother, my brother, and I moved to North Carolina. Maybe my apprehension about asking for a bathroom break (and my need in general to be seen as the good girl) resulted from my witnessing all the verbal fighting in the years leading up to my parents' split. There was too much important stuff going on in the adult world for me to complicate things with my mess ups. I vividly remember the feeling in that moment—the moment when my bladder was about to burst—of not wanting to put anyone out or disrupt the event if I could help it. There were already other kids doing that, and I wasn't going to add to the chaos.

Once I realized how badly that could turn out, I resolved to never again release my bladder outside of a bathroom. And so, our new life in North Carolina post-divorce started with a fresh set of challenges. While making friends was the surprisingly easy part of the transition to a new home state, my mounting phobias were not. I packed up my math bee experience and brought it with me to my next school. I was hell-bent on never finding myself standing in a puddle of my own pee.

My plan seemed to work perfectly until I was asked to stay for an after-school parent-teacher conference midway into the fall semester.

"I'm concerned about your daughter's health," Mrs. Williams told my mother. "Carrie asks to go to the restroom every thirty minutes, and this has been going on for weeks." Her face showed a mix of genuine concern and puzzlement. "Have you checked with her pediatrician to see if she has a bladder or kidney infection?"

This was news to my mother. After a doctor's visit and heart-to-heart conversation, my mother deduced that I was terrified of embarrassing myself again by losing control of my bladder. Going to the bathroom every thirty minutes, or fourteen times a day by Mrs. Williams's calculation, was how I took control. I was managing my fear quite well, thank you very much.

That traumatic stage-wetting event was also the turning point where the shy, meek, hide-in-the-shadows urge ended and the see-me-I'm-here compulsion took its place. Starved for attention stemming from the abandonment I felt when my father left to start another life, I began seizing every opportunity to put myself in the spotlight. I wanted to be seen, to be noticed, to be loved and adored—if not by my father, then by everyone else in my family.

The fifth issue stemming from my childhood actually started with my grand entrance into this world. I tell people that I came out of the womb hopping mad. (A wacky New Age explanation may be some sort of past life karma, perhaps?) As twisted as it sounds, I found security in this alter-ego. The tough, angry exterior showed the world exactly who was in control. I may appear petite and frail, all 105 pounds of me, but know my leopardess for ten seconds, and you'll see what she's capable of. And it is not always pretty. That fierce leopardess who later appeared to defend my precious pharmaceutical sales career at all costs reared her protective head throughout my childhood. She was always available to take control when circumstances felt unmanageable.

I think I must have learned early on that taking control was the only way to withstand the emptiness and insecurity I often felt inside. Taking control helped protect me from embarrassment, vulnerability, and shame. Exhibiting anger—yelling, fists in the air, raging—made me feel powerful in spite of my fears. Rage felt like control. My inner leopardess gave me strength. She gave me an identity that seemed to fill the half-empty cup that otherwise contained mostly self-rejection.

I cannot remember exactly when my intense perfectionism (basically control in a slightly different form) kicked in. It seemed to have followed me around like an attention-starved puppy as far back as I could remember. Perfectionism and anger—they were strangely addictive means of attaining a sense of control. There is a certain amount of comfort in the familiar, even if it is destructive.

My meticulousness seems to have hit an all-time high in my teens.

In junior high school, permed locks and feathered bangs channeled my creative energy. Every morning I turned my average hair into the perfectly sculpted work of art that rested upon my shoulders; this was both satisfying and incredibly maddening. I wanted desperately to be like everyone else, but I felt an equal pull to stand out, to be seen. My hairdo was my ticket to both.

All of my teenage angst was tied up in this elaborate morning ritual—brush out the knots, smooth the otherwise frizzy chemically-created curls (toxic rotten egg odor, notwithstanding), pull up just the right number of strands from both sides of my face and atop my head to come together in my tortoise barrette with a perfectly rounded dome. Then the hot curling iron created a tight lobster roll of hair that I would allow a few minutes to cool before teasing to bangs perfection. A slight irregular bump in the brushed dome, a stray hair that didn't make it into the barrette, or any lopsidedness perceived in the sculpting of my bangs just wouldn't do.

As my mother called me to breakfast the anxiety would intensify.

"Aaaaahhhh! Almost done. Just please leave me alone so I can concentrate!" I would scream in response, continuing the battle between my unruly hair and the plethora of beauty supplies in front of me.

Divots and paint chips peppered the inside of my bedroom door from the multiple occasions when I threw my brush against the molding, ultimately splitting the wood. The disfigured door seemed to serve as a constant reminder of my anger and my flaws. Attempting to fix those imperfections while feeling the pressure to get out the door on time and the intense need to look a particular way to both fit in and stand out was another example of how I let anger lead the way. In this case, it led the way to my missing the school bus yet again.

I loosened up in college a lot but not entirely. I figured I deserved a bit of a break from the college-preparatory pressure because I had been accepted by a good school, which was certain validation that I was worthy of love and acceptance. Those four years in college may have been the only time until very recently that I truly knew how to live in the moment. I was largely unfocused on the past and the future. I was able to experience so much of my time there in real time, only being pulled back into my irrational fears on occasion.

If freshman year spring break looked like something out of a bad reality TV show—twelve girls crammed into two rooms of a roadside motel in the panhandle of Florida living on wine coolers and fast food—sophomore year's was a somewhat tame frat party at my grandparents' beach house in North Carolina. My roommate and I were the lone females for most of the week, giving us a much-needed break from girl drama and evenings of playing dress-up for group dinners and bar crawls. We mostly stayed on the beach by day and in the house playing cards at night. It was the perfect college vacation . . . until it wasn't.

On the last night, someone suggested a bonfire on the

beach. While I was busy talking myself out of any legal concerns about defiance of beach rules, all the others were enjoying the sounds of the crashing Atlantic waves just beyond the warmth of the dancing flames. Little did I know that I would have to explain my way out of more than just some simple house guidelines if the cops showed up to smother the fire. As I joined the group, I realized that it had become a pot circle; I was not going to be able to wiggle my way out of this one easily. My first experience with cannabis was going to happen at my childhood vacation spot under the light of the moon, surrounded by friends I thought I trusted.

As the bong was puffed and passed, I followed suit with as much feigned nonchalance as I could. As I watched one after another falling like dominos into their mellow bliss, my mind kept analyzing why, after three or four rounds, I was feeling nothing. As my inner leopardess was about to express my frustration in such a way that would have me marching back to the house like a fed up toddler, one friend encouraged me to take more than my share of two puffs. So I took more. And more. My need to control the experience was on steroids, or drugs, as it were. I wish I could tell you what happened next, but that time has been erased for me. The next thing I remember was lying in the sand in fetal position, trying to understand why the world was spinning and all my friends were scattering like cockroaches away from the dampening flames of our little community bonfire.

One friend was kind enough to stay out there with me, and we somehow managed to make our way closer to the house. I froze and fell to the ground a few feet before the bottom of the staircase that would lead me to a comfortable bed and shelter from the increasingly cold breeze. That did not matter to me as much as the few blades of oat grass tightly woven in my grasp that kept me from flying away. I held on for dear life, convinced that if I relinquished my grip in the slightest, my body would be whisked up and into the foreboding midnight sky above.

My friend tried to ease my fears. He sat there beside me, holding my other hand, patiently waiting until he could gently nudge me slightly closer to the rest of the party that had been taken inside. But now, not only was I unwilling to let go, I had the strange sensation that my tongue was getting ever larger.

"My thongue feelths like a lemonnn," I told him, as I tried to open my mouth wide enough for him to inspect.

"It looks completely fine," he assured me. Fears of an anaphylactic reaction now set aside, I tried to wrap my mind around how I would be able to get through life unnoticed as my ever-expanding tongue got so big it would hang from my lips, sprout vines, and use my body as soil for an elaborate lemon tree. I continued to sit there for what seemed like hours until the creepy sensations wore off enough for us to hobble up one flight of stairs to the house and another up to my bedroom. As I lay in bed, I heard whispers of ridicule and laughter at my expense from the party below. I was the butt of their jokes.

I'm a disgrace. They all hate the freak that I've become—walking lemon tree and all, I thought as I finally let go enough to drift off to sleep.

A night's rest, a hearty breakfast, and a few self-depre-cating jokes the next day were all I needed to bounce back. But it would take me decades to understand that no, the pot was not laced with some sort of hallucinatory chemical. I just did not know how to let go of my insatiable need to control my body and everything around me.

@ @ @

There were plenty of blessings during my childhood too, though. When we moved to North Carolina, our cousins became our best friends. My aunts and grandparents came to be an instant tribe of elders who made me feel safe and loved. Attention felt glorious, and I quickly found myself drawn to being in the center of it. I would lead my younger cousins and brother in dramatic reenactments of popular commercials we filmed with a camcorder. They were always willing to follow my lead as director and head actress, play-ing various parts for the camera, day after day, week after week. Eventually, these childhood roles morphed into var-ious oratorical contests, debates, and theater productions, even landing me a starring role in eighth grade where I screamed as a heroin-addicted teen mother giving birth. In addition to fueling my budding creativity, I was gaining confidence and a can-do attitude.

Then there were negative consequences of those years that likely impacted my health in the long-term. When I wasn't commanding an audience to satiate my need to be seen, I was hyper-focused on controlling my surroundings. Like the constipation that kept my emotions (and painful stools) tightly bundled inside, protecting my body from a number of perceived harms gave me more ways to attempt to avoid discomfort. My concerns about losing control showed up in many ways when I was young: obsessive thoughts, anxiety about the house burning down, choking phobias. My fears were serious enough that I went an entire week without eating after learning about choking safety in fourth grade. When we learned about fire dangers the following month, I proceeded to check every outlet and appliance in the house before going to bed.

My number one fear for most of my life was puking. Emetophobia is the fear of vomiting, watching someone else vomit, seeing vomit, or even feeling nauseated. This started after a stomach bug at age six. Strangely, I only remember getting extra love and attention from my parents, but the fear was pronounced enough for my mother to use it to get me to stop biting my nails in second grade. My mother's convenient ruse involved painting my fingernails with no-bite polish. She said it was guaranteed to cause vomiting with the slightest touch to the mouth, and I believed her. It was years later that I realized it was plain ole clear nail polish. The fear of hurling far outweighed the anxiety-soothing benefits of biting my nails.

The uncanny ability to control myself kept me from blowing chunks for thirty-eight years of my life. On the surface, it may appear that I was simply afraid of the wretched (pun intended) act of puking. But in reality, I was scared of losing control. The antidote to that would have been to trust that my body is wise and knows when it needs to purge, surrendering to an experience shared by all living creatures.

For example, college and alcohol. I did as many socially awkward perfectionists do at that stage of life and finally let go a bit. I found myself partaking in volumes of alcohol that could tranquilize a horse. In the days following those nightly escapades, I was never seen in and out of the restroom like my friends. My body apparently did not understand how to detoxify from the alcohol properly, and at the slightest hint of functioning, willpower made it go away. Instead, I would endure two- or three-day hangovers in bed, but not once did I throw up.

Nor did I throw up during either of my pregnancies—even with morning sickness. Nausea was a constant fixture in both pregnancies. Relief by expulsion was not.

By the time my kids were young and stomach bugs became regular occurrences in our household, I had learned to stockpile anti-nausea medications whenever I could get them. Leftover from my pregnancies, check. Mother-in-law's surgery, check. Dad's colon procedure, check. It became my crutch; taking the antiemetic would ensure no loss of control in the form of upchucking. If the boys brought home a bug that made its way to me despite my best hygienic efforts, I would grip the sides of the bed, face and body drenched in sweat, squirming and moaning as if enduring some sort of exorcism until the wave of nausea subsided. Everyone else in the house would handle the occasional virus like a human. My fear of the unknown (vomiting) turned me into a rabid-looking animal.

My fears, strangely and perhaps unfortunately, brought me some comfort. My actions to avoid those earlier grade school obsessions that the house would burn down or I would choke to death helped me feel in control. Acting like Wonder Woman to claim victory in the fight against my nauseated body felt like strength and safety. If I could control my external environment, if my outer world was tidy, then my inner instability was not quite so scary.

Micro-managing fears by trying to control them wasn't an effective long-term solution, though. Eventually, I would have to learn to overcome them if I wanted to get out of this game of worry whack-a-mole. Overcoming fear took dedication and courage. It would require much of each to dredge up from the trenches both overt and hidden fears to investigate them thoroughly in the years to come. I had not yet connected the dots, but I would learn that it is by processing and moving through these fears that I would be able to heal my body.

Feeling safe is a primal urge, but I did not feel safe growing up. I did not feel a strong sense of predictability since disrupted routines had been my norm from the time I was born. When I was an infant and toddler my father was home for a while and then away for months. When I was a grade schooler and teen, weekends were spent being transported across state lines to visit the other caregiver while several romantic partners and eventually step-parents came into the mix. Divorce disrupts a child's understanding of family, and it led me to feel as if I was alone and unsure of my place in the world.

This need to control would continue to backfire—in more ways than one. Shortly after graduating college and sliding into a predictable bank job, I found myself in the waiting room of the only female ob-gyn my health insurance covered. I was relieved to be a patient of a doctor who actually possessed the anatomical parts she was examining. The whole nether area investigation scenario is too awkward with legs splayed in stirrups for me to be willing to see a male doctor. (Female ob-gyns are the norm now, but in the 1990s, only about twenty-two percent of them were female.) Unfortunately, I was not having those parts inspected this time. Nope. As much as I disliked those appointments, I would *rather* have been there for my annual exam. This visit, however, I needed someone to investigate my ass. I had constipation, straining, fissures, bleeding, you get the idea.

The doctor discovered that I had anismus, which is an inability to relax the anal sphincter muscle fully. Good stuff. My anus was basically a metaphor for my childhood. A product of divorce, I was unable to trust that anyone would be there for me. I was never able to relax in my pursuit of perfection. Now the issue had traveled from my head down to my anus, which could not loosen up either. Fortunately, this doctor had a solution for me: tight ass surgery.

The big day arrived, and as I sat in a triage room the size of a postage stamp awaiting the anesthesiologist, a nurse came in to top off my Fleet enema. Before I could even sit back up and find pieces of the doll-sized hospital gown to cover my backside, the young attractive sedation doctor came in to meet us. I soon learned he had attended Davidson College, the same liberal arts school from which I had recently graduated. What fun! To make this situation even more awkward, my enema was doing its job really well. The liquid had to come out of the hole from whence it came NOW. "Where's the restroom?" I asked, trying my best to appear casual as if my behind was not about to explode. The doctor replied, "Oh, just behind that curtain," meaning the curtain that was two feet from where we stood. There was no time left to find another bathroom, so I proceeded to relieve myself on the other side of a wispy curtain mere feet from my fellow Davidson alum. If he heard the explosive honks and vibrations, he did not acknowledge them, as I returned humiliated from behind the barely opaque room divider. That was considerate, I guess.

The surgery itself went well, except for the part where I awoke to order the surgeon to move his scalpel to the other side because he was not doing it right. Even under anesthesia I. Just. Don't. Let. Go. Surrender? Nope, wasn't really my thing. Control. Now *that* felt good.

If everything around me was under control—all three billion, four hundred thousand, thirty-five possible things were just right—then all was well. Did I even realize how exhausting that was? It was so obviously impossible to manage everything in my external environment and prevent potential discomfort in my internal world. But I did not see it that way. Control worked. It gave me something to hang on to—until it did not.

The solution to anismus was surgery, which went fine. But to correct my mind's trust issues and need for control, I would need more than a nip and tuck at the other end.

CHAPTER 4

Food as Medicine

BECAUSE I WAS STILL STRUGGLING WITH DIGESTIVE distress in my 30s, I tried new ideas wherever I could find them. In the fall of 2011, Amanda, the aesthetician I was visiting, told me how she cured her irritable bowel syndrome (IBS), and I was eager to learn more.

While I treated myself to a dermatologist-recommended microdermabrasion from her, Amanda detailed her erratic digestion. I related to the episodes of humiliation she described. I had experienced those random encounters with embarrassing digestive distress on more than one occasion.

When Amanda mentioned a book touting the benefits of a mostly alkaline diet—a regimen that promised increased energy, an end to digestive woes, and even noticeably clearer skin—I was already all in. The book claims that a diet high in acidic foods like meat, sugar, and processed foods leads to a detrimental pH balance in our tissues. Acidity in the tissues, according to the author, equates to poor health. To compensate for the excess acid, for example, some research suggests that the body could draw calcium from the bones. If you implement a few simple dietary changes, the author promises, your body, mind, and spirit will feel strong in a way that can never be achieved on the standard American diet. I considered the possibility. My energy could use a boost, I reasoned, and anything that could help my family's immune systems sounded good to me. Month-long stretches free of colds and stomach ailments were a luxury that we rarely enjoyed. This exciting new way of eating was worthy of consideration.

I have always tackled every challenge by learning as much as possible about it. Whether it was the latest drug I had to sell, a new community I was living in, or how to recreate a perfectly executed superhero birthday party, I read as much as I could, like I did with this new kind of medicine: healthy food.

I devoured the book Amanda recommended and resolved to take control of my body by taking control of my diet. The author explained that maintaining a proper pH, the acid versus alkaline balance in your blood and tissues, is an essential component to the overall health of our bodies. Tipping the scales toward the alkaline side by making specific food choices is the key to disease prevention, the book claimed. I was not fully convinced that my immune system was weaker than any other mom with two young kids bringing home a daily parade of germs, but I had a sense that my body was not as robust as it could be.

I forged ahead on this culinary healing adventure, converting myself and my family to a mostly vegan regimen of tofu steaks, vegan mayonnaise, and flaxseed baked goods. To achieve bodies primed for increased energy and vibrant health, I reduced our intake of acidic foods like meat, dairy, refined sugars, and faux food (the processed boxed and packaged stuff) and drank a morning glass of lemon water. It took me a bit to make sense of where different foods fall on the alkaline-acid spectrum, as some fruits that are acidic before consumed, like lemons, are alkaline to the blood and cells. This new diet did not offer a whole lot in the way of exciting meals, but I figured I could live without the joy of cooking and eating if it meant that I would be healthy and feel great.

My boys were young enough to try whatever I put in front of them, but when I made one particular mac n' soy-cheese a tad too heavy on the "cheese," seven-year-old Colin turned green and looked up at me with those compassionate eyes that said, "I'm sorry, mom, I just can't make myself like this one." The recipes required some tweaking, and once I learned that soy was not a good fit for my family, I managed to make meals that were at least palatable. I forged ahead, drinking lemon water every morning and serving meals devoid of meat, dairy, and processed foods.

It was not long after implementing the pH book recommendations that I began to notice the energy and vibrancy the author promised. My body, mind, and spirit did feel strong after I made those changes. I picked up running, something I had not done since college and had never enjoyed until now. I savored being able to breathe easily through my nose for the first time I could remember. It was early in our culinary adventure, but my immune system felt hearty with no hint of a cold after the germy, family-filled extended holidays. Rising early and tackling my days with vigor made me feel I could conquer the world, so I dismissed the two nights I awoke to nauseating stomach pains, which left me curled up on the bathroom floor. That I had eaten dinners rich in whole wheat pasta both of those evenings barely registered on my health radar. I explained away these blips thinking they were due to food poisoning or a passing virus. Up to this point in my life (other than my brief encounter with exhaustion during and after the birth of my first son), I had always been a bit of an Energizer Bunny, but this felt almost superhuman. Before long, I was touting the benefits of this lifestyle change to every mom and neighbor I knew.

"The secret is to significantly reduce your consumption of processed foods, meat, and dairy. Dairy has really been the life-changer for me," I excitedly told a friend as we watched our boys dive head-first into pathogen-infested plastic bricks. The birthday party of the week would have grossed me out in the past given our propensity for catching the latest round of sicknesses. But now, realizing my new level of stellar health, I was fearless. This party in particular was a dream for my Lego fanatic three-year-old, who had been known to leave the potty with toilet paper hanging from his backside to return to his latest medieval castle or small-town village creation.

"I mean, it's crazy that by changing what I eat I've been able to eliminate my sinus allergies and I have more energy than I've had in years. You've seen me running through the neighborhood, right? It's crazy. I'm not a runner!" I said with what I noticed felt like a hint of mania in my voice. My mind quickly brushed that thought aside, though, as I was on a high.

A relatively fit man wearing gym shorts smoothly approached us and joined the conversation. "I heard you talking about how diet has impacted your health," he started, as he wiped the peanut butter off his hand and then offered it in introduction. "I'm Chad. My son, Sawyer, is over there with the toddler-sized Lego crane. Loves anything having to do with construction. Which one's your son?" he asked.

"Bennett is the one in the 'My mom is my hero' hoodie in the back," I replied, laughing. "I'm taking full advantage of dressing him as long as he'll let me!"

I turned to introduce my neighbor, and she was nowhere to be found. She must have taken this opportunity to escape my infomercial. I guess I had mentally fabricated any hint of interest from her. *Oh well, it's not for everyone.*

"Have you changed the way you eat recently?" I asked, now that I had a captive audience.

He told me about the drastic measures he had recently undergone in an effort to reverse some alarming lab work. He said heart disease runs in his family, and he was not ready to succumb to a lifetime of medications to manage that same fate. So far, his efforts mostly involved ditching most of his packaged foods in exchange for whole foods.

"I haven't been back for follow-up labs yet," he said, "but I'm sleeping better and feel less sluggish. It seems like I'm on to something." I nodded in agreement. My body was electric, and its energy was leaving me giddy.

That school year, both kids had meanwhile been experiencing more than their share of stomach viruses. This was typical for elementary age children, we reasoned at first. But as the frequency increased, we began to get the sense that something was not quite right. Eventually seven-year-old Colin's sporadic stomach bugs developed into regular seizure-like vomiting spells. This happened at least a half dozen times about ten days apart. There seemed to be no apparent link, no specific food recently ingested, and no virus going around his classroom between the incidents. They came out of nowhere and were sometimes quite violent. Matt and I spent months carting Colin around to specialists, from the gastroenterologist to the neurologist at the children's hospital, trying to figure out the source. But all the appointments and tests we put him through did not determine a cause.

One day his school called for me to pick him up early from their classroom Thanksgiving celebration. When I arrived, his teacher pulled me aside, visibly concerned, and told me the events of the day. All the kids were gathered around for circle time after having devoured her much-anticipated homemade stone soup when Colin fell over, began trembling, and threw up on himself. When I arrived he looked a little weak, but largely the same healthy boy I had dropped off that morning. Though he recovered quite quickly, I think his teacher took a bit of a hit to her pride. Never before had her treasured soup taken a child down like that.

"I really, really did love your soup, Mrs. Sheen," Colin promised in that sweet little chipmunk voice of his as he took my hand and we left the room.

I began to think if attention to diet could heal me, maybe there was a nutritional answer for this, too. Now that major medical causes were ruled out and we remained stumped, I suggested we try an elimination diet. While our pediatrician maintained there was little clinical evidence that diet could be a contributing factor and that Colin likely contracted a virus that had simply been hanging around, my intuition told me something different.

I had been tinkering with eliminating foods from my own diet, so I considered trying a similar approach with my son. Through my reading and my most recent foray into the documentary *Forks Over Knives*, I learned even more about the evils of acidic meat—this time from an environmental and animal cruelty angle. I was making much of our food from scratch with natural, unprocessed ingredients that we could pronounce. I had also heard about a growing number of children and adults with gluten, dairy, and nut sensitivities. Now that it seemed we had exhausted all our mainstream medical options, I decided to eliminate all things dairy from his diet and fully removed them from mine, too. After all, my allergies had disappeared when we reduced our dairy intake, and I felt more energetic than ever because of it. Going a step further and completely eliminating it from our household was worth a shot.

Fortunately, Colin did not fight this much. Almond replaced the cow milk in his cereal, and I was able to find a coconut milk version of his favorite yogurt flavors. Cheese had never been his thing with the exception of pizza. We would tackle that potentially sticky situation later. Wouldn't you know it, the vomiting stopped. Two weeks went by and then two more. I found a recipe with coconut cream in lieu of dairy for his eighth birthday cake a few months later, and he continued to hold his food down.

Not long afterwards, our younger son, Bennett, followed in his big brother's footsteps. Again we thought maybe these vomiting episodes were a normal part of childhood. His pediatrician told me, "Their digestive tracts take time to develop; just manage the symptoms. They get through it." But as Bennett started throwing up every few weeks, I jumped into the solution that worked for his brother and removed all dairy from the house. This round was not quite as easy because this boy loved his Go-GURT, cheese sticks, and ice cream. With a little grocery store sleuthing, I converted my second child to a dairy-free diet as well. I swapped almond and coconut products for their dairy counterparts and even convinced him that the oil-concocted mozzarella-style vegan shreds made for an excellent grilled cheese. In time, my younger son's cyclical gastrointestinal (GI) distress subsided as well.

Wanting tangible proof that food is medicine, I found myself roaming the halls of the children's hospital with both boys this time. Instead of neurological exams and sleep studies for Colin's seizure-like vomiting, allergy tests for potential GI-inducing anaphylactic reactions, and gastroenterology consults for the possibility of chronic infections or parasites, I insisted that they check them for lactose intolerance and gluten sensitivity.

By the end of the long day spent waiting between blood draws and balloon-breathing tests with only Dora the Explorer and a few well-worn books to keep them occupied, the boys were being, well, brothers. As I was driving home amid the frequent meltdowns over snatched toys and spilled juice, I got the call.

"Good news, Mrs. Eckert. It looks like the boys are not lactose intolerant, and neither one has celiac disease."

I was stumped and hung up the phone with polite thanks and a resolve to make sense of what we were experiencing—not simply for my own inquisitive mind, but in preparation for the skepticism I was sure to face. Without definitive proof of a link, how could I possibly convince their other caregivers, like grandparents and family friends, that dairy was off limits for my boys?

But eliminating dairy did make a difference, I thought. *The boys have both stopped vomiting. Could it really have been this simple? Why then did the GI test results come up negative for lactose intolerance? And what about celiac disease? Does that mean we are in the clear? There is no need to consider tossing the wheat?* These were a few of the many questions that went unanswered at that point.

Test results aside, I thought, *the evidence is there for my boys and me.* Since we had cut out dairy, my seasonal allergies disappeared. The sinus congestion that had been a constant part of my life since I was a kid just went away, as did Colin and Bennett's vomiting. That was proof enough for me.

CHAPTER 5

Wired and Tired

WITH THE SUCCESSES OF MY SONS' COMPLETE RECOV-
eries, my own newfound energy, and my sinus health, I
continued to integrate the credo attributed to Hippocrates
into my lifestyle: Let food be thy medicine and medicine
be thy food. Given these positive results, I stuck with this
ride on the vegan bandwagon as we headed into 2012. I
figured a few dietary changes would be the answer to all
our future problems, and I stayed busy converting myself
and my family into the picture of health—one meatless,
dairy-free, plant-based meal at a time.

With my renewed energy, Matt and I visited our
shared dream of welcoming a little girl to our family. I
now felt robust enough to carry another child, and he was
thrilled. Let the baby-making commence once again! It
seemed that our dream of adding a baby girl to balance
the male energy in our household was not meant to be.
Sadly, I had an early miscarriage in December and then
stopped having periods entirely. My libido was suddenly

now tanked, and with conception out of the question, I was not interested in sex. Even if another pregnancy had been a possibility, I was back to fearing that my body could not handle the physical burden of carrying a child, much less being responsible for another life over the next eighteen years.

Around this time a weird pain in my hip flexor kept me from sitting on the floor to play Legos with my toddler and join my family for bike rides through the park. I never knew when the swinging of my leg to get on or off my bicycle might lead to a sharp twinge that would temporarily cripple me. I also found myself mildly nauseated most days. It felt like roiling waves of liquid were sloshing around in my stomach stuck mid-digestion. I ignored these minor inconveniences, though, because I was so thrilled with the energy I had regained once those pesky colds and allergy congestion were no longer dragging me down.

After a wonderful vacation with my husband to San Francisco in the spring of 2012, where we enjoyed a few fabulous vegan restaurants I had researched ahead of time, we came home to a five-year-old with a nasty virus, a respiratory illness with lingering effects that would alter my life for, well, forever. Everyone in the house caught it, but I took pride in being the least symptomatic and enduring only two days of fevers and an abundance of sleep. However, my energy never fully recovered, and after this point, I felt a mysterious decline of my body, part by part.

I cancelled spring break plans several weeks later, still too fatigued to host guests. Instead, I tried to entertain my kids on their week off, but I was bewildered that my malaise progressed into what I can best describe as mud-in-my-veins fatigue, mixed with dizzying brain fog, later doused with periods of intense anxiety. I felt disconnected from what was going on in the moment and had a surreal sensation of hovering outside my body while I attempted to tell my limbs how to slog through the heaviness of life.

As weeks went on, I found myself nodding off in the afternoon carpool line and sticking my kids in front of the TV after school so that I could take a nap. Yet I would typically wake up in the morning with so much energy I was almost manic. Hands shaking, heartbeat rapid, and a general sense of nervousness, I would emerge in dictator mode.

"Sit still. I need to fix your hair!" I commanded in the morning, restraining Bennett with one arm wrapped around his torso and the other reaching for the bottle of Fairy Tales conditioning spray we kept on the shelf above their backpacks. The daily ritual was my attempt to prevent them from ever coming home with head lice.

As I headed over to my other son, bottle of lice armor in my hand, I noticed Bennett raiding the pantry for the third time already this morning. "No more Goldfish," I said, slapping the package out of his grip and pulling his arm away from the door as I forcefully shut it. "You've had enough junk. Grab your lunch box and let's get out the door. Now."

As I dropped them off along the sidewalk beside the morning carline, I watched as Colin took Bennett's hand and guided him into the double doors of their elementary school. Now I was able to let my heart and mind linger for a moment. A lump began to form in my throat. The lump was filled with the acrid taste of guilt and regret. Why didn't I savor these moments with them? They would only be this innocent and sweet for a little while longer, and I was throwing away this precious time with my self-imposed edicts and militant rigidity.

It was as if suddenly the reality of life's steely morning demands stripped away the veil of peace and calm that had settled into me during the night's rest. My body could not adjust to the abrupt shift in existence. The energy made me productive in my work and household endeavors for a few hours but left me with little to give to my kids once their school day was over. This wired and tired, manic-then-crash roller coaster soon became my new norm.

On top of the energy fluctuations, my hip flexor pain got so bad that bike rides and missing Pilates sessions became the least of my worries. Eventually, I had to ever so carefully step in and out of the car to avoid the familiar tweak of torture. I started seeing a physical therapist, then a chiropractor, followed by an orthopedic surgeon, then another PT. I had an MRI, the results of which were vague and could have belonged to anyone's hip—frozen or completely functional. Many months and thousands of dollars later, my mysterious locked-up hip was still in pain. I felt like I was falling apart, and no one could figure out why or how to stop it.

My fatigue hit an all-time low one evening on our wedding anniversary when my husband cooked a lovingly prepared plant-based meal, the plate filled with perfectly roasted asparagus, peppers stuffed with quinoa and black beans, and artisan French bread.

"What a beautiful dinner. Thank you for all your hard work, honey," I said with all the enthusiasm and energy I could muster. I took a few bites and then proceeded to fall asleep at the dinner table—without even having a sip of wine.

◎ ◎ ◎

Baffled by my complete loss of energy and the cessation of monthly menstrual cycles that year, my primary care doctor encouraged me to look for an endocrinologist. The idea made sense. Maybe my lack of periods, unrelenting fatigue, and increasing digestive challenges had something to do with a hormone imbalance. It was a long shot, but perhaps my mysterious hip flexor pain was somehow tied up in this as well. My hormones had seemingly gone rogue and I needed to find someone to help me reign them back in.

One morning I was scrolling through our healthcare provider's website in my home office where, despite my ever-failing body, I enjoyed a few hours of creativity designing stationery for online clients. As I progressed to the second endocrinologist on my list, I felt an instant bond with the scheduler who answered my call. When I described my early miscarriage last December and my concerns about my menstrual cycle, she responded, "Well, honey, I would be exhausted too if I hadn't had my period for nine months! You're only 37?! We've got to get you in here ASAP!"

We then proceeded to share our experiences with nutrition as a means of healing. I could just see her sympathetic head nodding in agreement from her desk across town. *She really gets me,* I thought. Appointment booked, I hung up the phone feeling optimistic. We were going to figure this thing out. My hormones seemed to be at the root of my fatigue, and once the doctor regulated them, I figured, I would be back to my usual energetic self. Thyroid, adrenals, estrogen . . . they must be the source of all this craziness, and I was headed to find a solution with an expert of all things hormonal.

I had had a few weeks to do some more research on my apparent ailment, so on the day of the appointment, I arrived fully prepared. Thanks to my internet research I was now ninety-nine percent certain that I had something called adrenal fatigue, along with a possible thyroid imbalance. If, for some reason, the adrenal fatigue thing did not get his attention (because I had read that not all mainstream specialists recognize this diagnosis) then I would insist that he do a test for Addison's disease, a condition where your body does not produce enough of certain hormones. *I'm a smart woman,* I told myself. *I have done my homework. This is going to be a fantastic conversation.*

When the doctor entered the room, we exchanged quick pleasantries and then dove right into my symptoms, starting with my fluctuating fatigue and hip flexor pain.

"I also seem to go from being anxious with a rapid heartbeat to completely exhausted. There's no middle ground. Oh, and my digestion. I've been getting intense stomach cramps occasionally that wake me up at night." It was a mouthful, but I felt a rare boost of energy as the anticipation of a treatment path for a legitimate illness grew.

He looked at my thyroid numbers and immediately indicated that they were off. "Hypothyroid," he said, dismissively, not even looking up from his prescription pad to meet my gaze. This man's bedside manner was atrocious. I could not have felt more ashamed of my silly health complaints, moaning about my issues which he must see all the time. He explained that the reference ranges used by specialists are often narrower than those dictated to primary care physicians, and therefore he considered my numbers outside the normal range.

"Does that mean I have Hashimoto's thyroiditis, or is it an iodine deficiency?" I asked, wanting to impress him with my knowledge on the subject and restore some of the pride that was stripped when I realized that my problems were not unique. I desperately wanted him to *see* me.

"I had an iodine test, and the results showed that I'm low," I offered. "The thyroid needs iodine to function properly, right? From what I understand, most of us are deficient in iodine. It's weird, though, because when I had the MRI for my hip, I developed a reaction to the iodine. Does that mean I need more or less?" In just a few minutes, I had gone from energized to manic. And even though it felt as though I was talking to a wall, I continued.

"And what about my adrenals? Could they have something to do with my fatigue? I mean, I'm just so exhausted! Well, maybe not right at this moment. This is unusual. Must be because I'm in a different environment, and I'm actually getting help. I'm so relieved!" Despite my distress, this doctor could not even be bothered to look me in the eye and acknowledge my concerns. I felt like just another middle-aged mom with hormonal fluctuations and the expected mental imbalances that came along with them. I was not mentally imbalanced, I reasoned. Some very stable part of me was buried underneath this physically fragile and paranoid facade.

The doctor stared through me as though I did not really exist, then responded simply, "No. And I'm going to start you on a low dose of Synthroid."

No? What the hell does that even mean? I thought, deflated and agitated at the same time.

"But I don't do very well with medications. I'm very sensitive," I said. I have always needed less than the minimum dose of medications. I used to get wired on Sudafed growing up, and a simple cup of coffee tends to make me easily agitated. "Are you sure this is a low dose?" I had read something about a more natural thyroid replacement medication, but I couldn't remember what it was called, and this man seemed so displeased with me and all my research that I clammed up. I froze.

"Yes, I'm writing you a prescription for a low dose. Take it for three weeks, and then we'll follow up," he said, and walked out of the room.

That was it. I stood there, dumbfounded at his terseness. Then I swiftly got my act together, patched up the little hole in my deflated ego, and made a choice to embrace this healing journey. *It's a treatment path, right?* I reasoned. *My blood work is abnormal, and the doctor has a solution. I'm going to be okay.*

Two days into my baby dose of Synthroid, which I had chosen to split into quarters, I was a jittery, anxious mess. My heart was beating out of my chest, and my emotional combustibility was dangerously high. Sure, I had energy, but at what expense? *At least I will not fall asleep in car line again,* I thought as I navigated my way through traffic.

The feeling of intense fatigue was now replaced by the sensation that I was on some sort of cheap energy drink. My all-too-familiar road rage, likely picked up from my father, who routinely yelled expletives while driving when I was a kid, was dangerously close to surfacing, and the Synthroid only added fuel to the fire. When there is a cluster of cars in front of me that I cannot force my way through or someone is taking far too long to make a right-hand turn off a busy road, I feel trapped. I spew comments like, "Move over already!" "How can you hang out like that in the left lane going twenty-five miles an hour?" and "They should never have allowed you to get a license—idiot!" As soon as I can break free from the barricade, my mind and body feel free again, at least until I run up behind the next clump of vehicles.

One afternoon it was so bad I called the doctor's office from the car. The nurse suggested a lower dose and encouraged me to give it at least two weeks. *Uh, I can't go much lower than the mini-dose I've taken the liberty of choosing for myself,* I thought but did not say.

"The side effects should go away in a few days," she assured me.

A few more days turned into more than a week, and I was driving my family and myself crazy with my constant agitation. When I am agitated, I feel out of control, and I try to direct everything around me. My surroundings should be tidy; sounds must be muted; the temperature needs to be carefully regulated. Trying to live comfortably inside my home with two exuberant little boys running around while attempting to manage a household with mountains of toys and mounds of laundry seemed next to impossible.

"You're not the boss of me!" Bennett screamed one day after taking a hefty chunk out of Colin's arm with his mouthful of baby teeth.

"Maahm! Ben bit me again. I didn't do anything to him. It was my turn with the iPad!" Colin screamed back. I was more concerned with why my five-year-old was still biting.

Does he need therapy? Is this normal at his age? What if he does this at school one day? I thought. *How am I supposed to manage this behavior when I can't even get a grip on my own?*

Instead of pushing through the Synthroid, I decided to stop altogether and request to see a different doctor in the practice. I had hoped a female physician would have a bit more compassion. This time I had done research to arm me with mainstream terminology. Adrenal fatigue is largely ridiculed by allopathic medicine, the name given to the classic diagnosis and treatment of illness symptoms with medications or surgery. So I made sure to find a diagnosis with an ICD-10 code used by doctors and health insurance companies to represent a diagnosis, thus deeming it a "true" disease. I was planning to use the Addison's disease angle. Once I had finally managed to dig deep enough in my online searches to strike gold with this medically recognized disorder I was thrilled. It was a rare condition, but it was hopefully legit enough to get this new doctor's attention.

I learned that hypocortisolism, or Addison's disease, is a condition in which one's adrenal glands do not produce enough hormones, namely cortisol and aldosterone. Cortisol helps the body respond to stress and assists in maintaining blood pressure, heart function, the immune system, and blood glucose levels. Aldosterone is responsible for balancing sodium and potassium in the blood, which affects the amount of fluid the kidneys remove as urine, essentially regulating blood volume and blood pressure.

This diagnosis seemed to fit. I was not responding to stress well, evidenced by my recent bouts of anger and constant irritability. My blood pressure was low, and dizzy spells had become the norm when I stood up. And my immune system? Even though I did not catch anything when the rest of the family was sick, I was instead endlessly tired and moody. Intuitively, I felt that my immune system had gone offline and was no longer protecting me. Time was ticking, and if someone or something did not pull me from the sinking vehicle, I felt, I was going to drown. I was getting adept at backseat driving my mounting medical diagnoses, so it looked like I was going to have to save myself. Science and logic had always gotten me out of sticky situations in the past, and I was convinced that there was an answer out there for me this time as well. I felt I was onto something big.

"Carrie? Carrie? Is there a Carrie E. out here?"

That was my cue. It was my turn to meet this new doctor and plead my case. I was taken back to the same room in which I had sat a little over a month ago. I felt confident that this time would be different.

My new female endocrinologist entered the room, and within seconds any hope that I had managed to scrape back together with this newest bit of research disintegrated. She had less bedside manner than the previous doctor. Instead of shared female understanding, I sensed disdain. It seemed my complaining would only make me weaker in her eyes, so instead I kept details to myself and got straight to the point. "The Synthroid made me wired. I think I have Addison's disease," I said matter-of-factly. I sat up straight and tall to offset in outward confidence what sitting on this paper-covered exam table with my legs swinging like a child stole from my dignity.

"That's a major diagnosis," she said skeptically. "From what I see in your chart that's not the case." Again, zero eye contact, her head down, pen scribbling away on her clipboard. As my medical chart continued to expand with each office visit, I imagined what notes were being passed from doctor to doctor. My attempts at finding my own answers to my ailments probably branded me a problem patient. "Give this other medication a try," she urged, and that was it.

I left the office with a prescription for a new thyroid medication and a chastisement for giving up so hastily. On the way out the door I tossed the prescription in the wastebasket and vowed to investigate further.

I came away from this experience with a sense that an abnormal thyroid reading was only one small piece of a larger puzzle, and I was not interested in using a stopgap treatment with multiple side effects to manage something that needed a higher level of care.

CHAPTER 6

Environmental Toxins

THE HOT AND HEAVY FLORIDA CLIMATE WE HAD been living in for the past seven years kept us inside for much of the warmer months. But the weather was not the only factor preventing us from enjoying the outdoors. We also had to contend with the smoke from intermittent controlled burns just a few miles from where we lived. I would often feel the urge to yank my shirtsleeve up to cover my mouth as I made the short walk from the front door to the car. I would rush our dog, Maddie, to do her canine business quickly so that we could go back inside to the purity of our indoor air. Common sense told me it must not be a good idea to hang around in the haze and potentially impede my lungs further. I had enough physical issues to contend with already.

It seemed as if every few weeks the fire teams started another air-polluting blaze that created clouds of smoke outside our door whenever the wind blew in the right direction. I've always been inquisitive and I tend to question anything that gives me pause. Questions require answers. In this case, I couldn't help but wonder if they really had to do controlled burns and so I sought to find an explanation. Google told me that prescribed burns are crucial, especially in planned communities like ours, for the diversity of plant and animal life. It also reduces dead branches and debris that can fuel intense wildfires. These man-made burns help control invasive species and allow native plants that thrive upon burned remains to come back to life.

These low intensity burns and their inescapable odor got me thinking about the quality of the air we breathe and potential environmental toxins that enter our bodies through our lungs and skin. At this point in my health journey, I was relying on online research and a handful of books on healthy eating and environmental toxins. The website for the Environmental Working Group (EWG) was especially informative. After stumbling upon their Clean Fifteen and Dirty Dozen lists to help guide my produce purchases, I learned that just buying organic was not going to be enough to keep my family safe. I discovered that the dangers of such health bandits as estrogen-imitating BPA (the industrial chemical bisphenol A found in many plastics) and thyroid-altering organophosphate pesticides are all around us. Being mindful of using BPA-free plastics and consuming organic produce was a start. The more I dug into the research, the more overwhelmed I became with the knowledge that an endless amount of toxins were permeating our living environment. It seemed my steep learning curve was like a climb up the side of a mountain.

Most troubling to me was finding that the treatment techniques used to sanitize tap water vary significantly from state to state, leaving many of us to ingest unsafe levels of everything from known carcinogens to toxic chemicals and heavy metals. In Florida, hurricanes and storms cause floods that send contaminants like fertilizers into the water systems, making it one of the ten worst states for drinking water. The unsafe levels of copper and lead found in our water were surprising, but I was even more disgusted to learn about the coliform from human waste I was drinking. A reverse osmosis water filter eventually became a must-have in our kitchen.

Learning that drinking water across our country was not necessarily safe was just the crest of a whole new wave of health hazards I was uncovering in my home. I learned that carbon monoxide from gas stoves like ours can cause wheezing and increased sensitivity to allergens in those with asthma if not properly ventilated and monitored. Carpets and draperies can capture and retain any number of indoor allergens if not cleaned regularly with HEPA (high-efficiency particulate air) vacuum filters and air purifiers. To live in a healthy home, we would have to reduce our reliance on modern conveniences like plastic containers, Teflon, anti-bacterial soaps, artificial fragrances, and chemicals in new carpets and upholstery. It was overwhelming.

◎ ◎ ◎

I began to see the larger picture of dangerous environmental toxins infiltrating our modern world when I visited my favorite self-care hangout one day in 2012: the hair salon.

I checked in at the counter, grabbed the latest issue of *Real Simple*, and settled into the cushiony leather chair to wait for my stylist.

I was here to treat myself to highlights and was looking forward to the hair wash and relaxing temple massage. As much as I wanted to bask in the experience, though, the start of a knot was forming in my belly. In retrospect, that was probably a hint to give this hair care treatment a bit more consideration. Unaware of what that sensation meant, I swiftly dismissed it as something I had eaten that was not sitting well.

We discussed the logistics (the color to be applied, how much length to take off, etc.) and then dove into our usual catch-up chat. Talking about my latest ailments had become my preferred conversation starter. As I updated her on my recent doctors' visits and research into environmental toxins, I stared at myself with a head full of aluminum foil and became aware of a headache and slight dizziness settling in.

Maybe it was psychosomatic, but with my new knowledge of the toxins in so many products we take for granted as safe, I thought, *No wonder I felt like I had to drag my ass out of bed after my previous color treatments!* Not only had I breathed the chemicals as my hairdresser applied them, but my body had likely absorbed some of the dye. And I had spent night after night with my face pressed up against the freshly processed strands of hair. I realized this would be the last time I subjected my body to this noxious burden.

Ethanolamine, resorcinol, and p-phenylenediamine are

three common ingredients in hair dyes, I subsequently learned from reading articles posted on the EWG website. These ingredients have been linked to everything from respiratory and skin irritations to cancer and endocrine disruption. The list of ingredients in these products can be as long as a privileged American child's Christmas list, and with a significant lack of regulation in the beauty care industry, there is little ingredient transparency. The more I read, the more I learned that I was playing a game of chance anytime I applied a commercial beauty product.

If this class of chemicals could wreak such havoc on my endocrine system, then how could environmental toxins, like glyphosate (a common pesticide), building materials, and gas emissions possibly have been affecting the health of my body? It dawned on me that my family and I had likely been exposed to a few hefty loads of specific offenders in recent months.

Earlier that year, we had undergone a small construction project to convert our screened porch to an indoor air-conditioned space. The subcontractor on the project had overestimated the amount of concrete necessary, which required that they go back in and sand down the dry floor a few days later. Up to that point, my family had been living around the contained mess. The area was taped and tarped. And other than being a bit noisy at times, the construction had been mostly out of our way, so on the day of the sanding, I had not expected that to change.

That day my springer spaniel, Maddie, lay at my feet in the upstairs guest room/office while I worked at my computer. My preschooler, Bennett, babbled to himself happily in the adjoining space as he created his latest Lego village. When the noise of the sanding got too loud, I closed our doors and we continued to work and play unaware that anything was amiss.

About an hour later, I began to notice dust coming up into the room from under the closed door. When I opened it, I was blinded by a massive cloud of gray. My mama bear instincts kicked in as I surveyed my options—stay here and call for help or make a run for it. With the dust getting increasingly heavy and no possibility of getting the machine operator to hear me over the deafening whirl of his motor, I grabbed the blankets off the guest bed and wrapped up my son. Toddler in a blanket burrito on my hip and dog held by a belt-turned-leash, the three of us made a run for it. As I was shutting the front door behind us, I saw the loose panel of tarp flapping in the breeze.

The next day I got busy investigating concrete, and I found that most of the research on cement dust has focused on the long-term effects on construction workers and has indisputably concluded that their lungs take a dire hit. Lime, crystalline silica, and chromium found in this dust may also enter into the bloodstream, potentially reaching all the organs of the body. The microstructure and physiological performance of the heart, liver, spleen, bone, and muscles are most likely affected to some degree. Even if we were not the ones out there grinding the cement every day, the inside of our house was doused by dust that could linger in the air conditioning system. Concerned for our safety, I continued to research these ugly toxins.

Renovation construction is a different animal than new home construction, I learned. More precautions like thick, sealed tarps and exhaust ventilation need to be taken when residents occupy the home. The revelation that this construction mishap may have also played a role in my ailing health left an emotional rock of guilt, remorse, and shame in the pit of my stomach.

How could I have been so naive? How could I have thrown my children in harm's way? I thought. I was resigned never to make such a stupid mistake again.

CHAPTER 7

Gut Instincts

WITH THE FAILED SYNTHROID EXPERIMENT BEHIND me and a home toxin cleanup underway, I decided that being my own medical scientist was no longer cutting it. After nine months of veganism, my intuition told me it was time to see a nutritionist. Up to that point, I had been trying to make the plant-based diet work for me. It had led to such exuberance for a few months in late 2011, but then I crashed and never fully recovered from that pre-spring break respiratory virus in 2012. It had seemed so apparent that changing my diet was the golden ticket to vibrant health, but now I was beginning to wonder if it was that simple.

After a lengthy discussion regarding my symptoms and health history, the nutritionist suggested that my digestive tract was likely too compromised to break down and properly absorb the nutrients in a diet based on plants (often raw) and encouraged me to think about more of a Paleo approach to eating. As she explained it, something called

71

intestinal permeability, known also as leaky gut, was presumably to blame for the inflammatory immune response effecting not just my gut but possibly my thyroid as well.

The theory was that large protein molecules were getting into my bloodstream, where they were not supposed to be, due to the breakdown of the otherwise tight junctions of my intestinal wall. Apparently, you do not even have to be aware of gut symptoms to have leaky gut, so it was not surprising that this presumed diagnosis had been overlooked on my quest for sustained energy. Furthermore, the clinician argued that the sad state of my digestive tract—which manifested as unaddressed life-long constipation—could be caused by years of exposure to chemicals and food "toxins" like gluten.

Add back all the acidic meat? Eliminate the oatmeal, pasta, and bread to which I had grown accustomed? It felt like a reversal. I had started to give into cravings I could not seem to ignore by eating eggs and fish in moderation, but the thought of red meat now made my stomach churn. Maybe she was right; perhaps veganism was not working for me anymore. Maybe it would again down the road when my apparently damaged gut healed. I still had a lot of experimenting to do.

It suddenly dawned on me that those nights curled up on the bathroom floor after having eaten big bowls of healthy durum wheat pasta months ago might have had something to do with a sensitivity to gluten. I decided to take things one step at a time and first eliminate the gluten. This meant exchanging my whole wheat bread and pasta for rice-based, gluten-free alternatives. *Not so hard,* I thought.

Within days, my energy started to return. I was thrilled, but even then did not realize how strong that gluten connection was. After a few weeks, I began to allow myself a bit of gluten here and there. I would sneak a bite of a brownie made with spelt flour or enjoy traditional oatmeal (not inherently gluten-filled but problematic due to wheat cross-contamination and the widespread use of glyphosate), and my energy would plummet hard. I finally realized that there was likely a strong connection between gluten and both my fatigue and those agonizing middle-of-the-night GI flares I had experienced.

With the realization that something as simple as gluten could have such a detrimental effect on my digestion and having heard the buzz about the gut-brain connection, I naturally felt the pull to explore how I could heal my body's "second brain." The science was showing that intestinal distress could be both the cause and effect of anxiety, depression, and brain fog. The two organ systems are intricately linked and constantly in communication with one another.

As summer turned into fall, I decided to embark on a Gut and Psychology Syndrome (GAPS) protocol with a specialist in California. The GAPS diet, created by Dr. Natasha Campbell-McBride, focuses on healing and sealing the intestinal lining, or leaky gut, by consuming a limited number of nutrient-dense, easy-to-digest foods including meats, fish, egg yolks, fermented foods, and specific vegetables. I had seen this diet mentioned by a few healthy food bloggers battling various autoimmune challenges. The bloggers were healing (or seemed to be based on their slick websites and healthy social media following), so I did a little online digging and found a reputable practice willing to work with me remotely.

My laborious protocol was somewhat similar to the gluten-free, dairy-free, meat-filled diet I had adopted already but with more restrictions, including *all* grains, starchy vegetables, refined carbs, and egg whites. The process kicked off with a weekend of only chicken soup, during which I was hit with fevers, chills, nausea, and bread cravings so intense I was ready to raid the closest steakhouse for their buttery yeast rolls. My practitioner assured me this was an expected part of the process as my body rid itself of toxins. When I eased into solid foods again a few days later, she instructed me via our weekly phone calls and morning check-in emails to incorporate daily bone broth. Further into the process she added to my already overflowing pill cabinet customized supplements, including a probiotic to provide beneficial bacteria along the GI tract, fermented cod liver oil for the multiple benefits of essential fatty acids, juicing to naturally cleanse the liver, and digestive aids for proper elimination and liver support.

As if the food preparation and management of supplements were not challenging enough, I was growing weaker and more encumbered by the day. I had lost ten pounds and felt dizzy all the time.

"Why do you trust this GAPS woman again?" Matt asked me one day a few months into the protocol. "I mean, you haven't even met her in person. She can't see what this is doing to you!"

"I know this is good for me somehow," I said, but eventually realized I was losing this fight. My fatigue was worsening. My husband was beginning to worry for my life now that I had writhed in sweaty flu-like agony for days during the kick-off chicken soup fast and later embarked upon the accompanying iodine-loading protocol that sent me into a similar feverish delirium. I did believe this diet had its benefits. In fact, my research had convinced me that it was an excellent protocol for restoring balance to a badly damaged gut. Maybe I was just taking things too quickly and without the support I truly needed. Accepting any support (social or even medical) was not so easy for me given my self-sufficient approach to life (note the 2,000 mile distance between me and my chosen care provider).

I gave GAPS a really good shot and I was as meticulous a client as any nutritionist could ask for. Eventually I sensed that it was not going to be the answer I needed. Practitioners claim that the diet can take up to two years to heal the gut and even reverse autoimmune diseases, but after four months, this did not seem like the optimal route for me.

In working with my GAPS practitioner and reading about others who had gone through food-as-medicine and tailored supplementation protocols, I understood that deep healing often included uncomfortable detoxification side effects. The path to healing is not always smooth sailing. I felt confident that this protocol allowed for some significant gut repair and paved the way for the next step in my healing process. Now, though, I needed to dig further into the cause of my health challenges.

A perplexing year finally behind me, I felt a cautious sense of hope as I tiptoed into 2013. This newfound optimism was rekindled by a serendipitous introduction to a functional medicine internist, Cynthia Li, MD. My brother worked with Dr. Li's husband in northern California, and while chatting over dairy-free eggnog and grass-fed steak at a holiday party, he found an eerie number of similarities between her health journey and mine. When he told me about this physician who also personally experienced many of my same issues and was lost in her own "medical system" for years looking for answers, I decided to give her a call.

As she explained to me, functional medicine is a new paradigm that expands upon conventional Western medicine, focusing on root causes of chronic conditions instead of addressing downstream effects or managing symptoms. Increasingly more common, practitioners with functional medicine training use this root cause-based approach like detectives, sleuthing out the whys of disease—imbalances in hormones, the gut, the brain, the heart, immunity and detoxification ability—and more importantly, the hows of healing. This new paradigm of medicine is not only appreciated, it is critical.

I had now tried a plant-based pH diet, a mainstream medicine endocrinology route, a gluten-free mostly Paleo regimen, and a strict GAPS protocol. The intermittent symptom relief had felt more like a physical and emotional roller coaster ride. I sensed I needed someone with a broader body-mind perspective to help me navigate a new course. Dr. Li agreed to take me on as a patient, and with her guidance, I began to get to the root of my illness.

After filling out an extensive medical history and an hourlong video consultation, she explained that my body was chronically inflamed, likely caused by years of living in a fight-or-flight state. Myriad stressors—from environmental toxins to poor food quality to my high-achiever mentality—had taken a toll on my body's ability to unwind and balance my nervous system. When the nervous system is not given ample time to rest, it lacks the resources it needs to heal and becomes ripe for the development of dis-ease. Given my history with leaky gut and chronic inflammation, she suspected some sort of autoimmunity. As much as I had sought a diagnosis (in part to prove this sickness was real), she surprisingly did not want to box me into one if it was not necessary—patients can get identified with labels that can, in and of themselves, limit the potential to heal. The goal was to get to the root of my health challenges and to support my body's systems so I could heal myself. I did not, then, have to live with the name of an autoimmune condition that may or may not exist.

Upon listening to my dietary successes and woes of the past year and reviewing lab work, she designed a more flexible diet for me—one that was not dictated by the latest named and branded trends but one that felt more intuitive. Years later, she told me she had recognized the meticulousness of my dietary and supplement regimens as a pattern that patients often follow that can sabotage their healing: the stress of trying to do everything perfectly. At the time, however, she just recommended I focus on eating an abundance of organic fruits and vegetables, nuts/seeds, gluten-free grains, and some humanely-raised meat and fish, basically the way generations have grown up eating in the Mediterranean. She wanted me to be patient as I reintroduced foods outside my GAPS diet. Using my body as my guide, she advised me to pay attention to reactions such as energy fluctuations, mood changes, and skin and digestive problems each time a new food was added. For the first time in years, I felt that I was given permission to listen to my body instead of following a list of dos and don'ts. Growing up in a society that values outward appearances and measurable goals, it felt strange to lean into my felt senses instead of my mind for direction.

We spent the next several months tinkering with my food repertoire and weaning off some of my many supplements, a hodgepodge of pills compiled from the advice of various practitioners and my own online research. She wanted to significantly simplify my regimen, "which in and of itself can be a stressful load for your body," she told me. I could not tell what the iodine and ox bile were doing anyhow. With so many moving pieces, no one could tell if one particular pill was making my heart race or a certain food was blocking up my bowels. I was still as tired as I had been for almost a year, and it was like I was on a symptom seesaw. Reduce potential bodily stressors? That sounded good to me.

Until working with Dr. Li, I had not fully recognized the level of toxicity we had inhaled with the smoke from the controlled burns and the renovation dust in our home from the previous year. As she began telling me about the dangers of indoor air pollution, I realized that my gut had been right all along. Formaldehyde, mold, and possibly even mercury can linger in the trapped air of modern homes. Living in Florida, we do not get as many days where we can open our windows as homeowners in more moderate climates. Dr. Li armed me with a laundry list of healthy home tips like adding air-cleaning houseplants to every room, installing a filtered water system, using a HEPA vacuum, and removing carpets in lieu of wood or tile when possible.

Surprisingly, Dr. Li also prescribed daily relaxation/meditation practices including a 20-minute walk outside in nature. "Being in nature has been shown in research to stimulate the parasympathetic nervous system helping to decrease stress and allowing the body to rest and digest," she told me through the screen of a follow-up video appointment in January of 2013. The internet connection stalled for a moment and, instead of staring awkwardly at her frozen face and half smile, I looked at the room behind her. She appeared to be working from a home office. I could see a cozy bedroom darkened by closed draperies in the corner and a thick wool blanket strewn over a rocking chair to her right.

"Engage multiple senses: walk barefoot, smell a pinecone, touch a flower petal. These sensory activities will increase the parasympathetic response," she continued, holding her hands up and rubbing her fingertips to her thumbs to suggest a tactile experience. These recommendations seemed so simplistic. How much good could they really do to help me regain my strength and lessen my pain?

"If you're able, try to break a small sweat during the walk. If this makes you more tired afterwards, decrease your exertion the next time." Breaking a small sweat would be pretty simple considering most of my walking felt like battling quicksand. Much of the time Matt was there by my side giving me a sturdy arm to hold on to. The nature part sounded nice in theory, but the weariness I felt in the depths of my bones was screaming otherwise.

The bed is so much more comfortable. Please don't make these sand-filled legs move any more than they absolutely have to, my body whined in rebellion.

Following her advice by adjusting my dietary protocol over the next several months to more loosely follow a whole foods approach, I sensed that my gut was healing. Since fatigue was my main symptom, and it lingered, it was hard to know for sure. If nothing else, I was learning to trust my gut when it came to making food choices instead of relying on a dietary list of rules. This was, however, not as easy as it sounds. For decades I had followed my gut's lead by feeding its sugar cravings, pulling up to the nearest drive-through at the first twinge of a hunger pang, and offering it any number of antacid, anti-nausea, or anti-bloating medications if it didn't feel good. Wasn't I "trusting my gut" then? I was getting the sense that a deeper level of intuition had to be a part of the equation for this avenue to be successful. Tuning into more subtle bodily cues, that weren't always overtly GI related, was my new approach. The more I became mindful of my eating and curious about a food's aftereffects, the more I was aligning with my body.

I eventually felt that it was time to incorporate detoxifying and cleansing green juices, sea vegetables, algae, and raw vegetables into my diet. The benefits of fresh, raw vegetables have never been lost on me. I was malnourished, and my gut was compromised from decades of poor food choices and lifelong stress. I had learned from my GAPS practitioner months ago that a robust and healthy gut, once rebuilt with nourishing foods first, is crucial for digestion of these cleansing raw vegetables.

I began implementing all of Dr. Li's lifestyle recommendations right away, but I put most of my effort into perfecting the food going into my belly. I soaked and sprouted nuts to improve their absorption potential; I fermented cabbages, cucumbers, and carrots to feed my gut with beneficial bacteria; and I immersed myself in the vast online world of grain-free recipes and the intricacies of cooking lean grass-fed meat. Not surprisingly, these tasks consumed me, and true to my nature, I wanted to take control of each ingredient I ingested.

CHAPTER 8

Embrace Your Grace

AS 2013 PROGRESSED AND I CONTINUED TO SEEK solutions to so many unanswered questions about my health, manifestations of my dis-ease evolved as well. In addition to a locked hip, a cessation of monthly periods, fatigue that had me glued to the sofa much of the time, and an endlessly chattering mind, I found myself struck by unusual migrating pains—a sensation in my forearm that oscillated between numbness and throbbing or shoulders so tight I could barely turn my head to see my children in the back seat of the car.

Thankfully, my seasonal allergies and monthly colds had ceased, but in their place came a plethora of bewildering issues. My body rarely felt at ease, especially in stillness. Sitting on the sofa to watch TV with my family meant I would have to continually attempt to distract my mind from the stabbing pain in my lower back, the rock in my neck that seemed to crack and crumble with any head movements, and the numbness in my arms that crept in if they stayed motionless too long. I usually ended up decamping to the floor—either working through some yoga poses I had learned from classes at the local studio or creating a bed for myself on the carpet. Lying down was easier than sitting.

Those floating pains were now labeled as fibromyalgia on my medical charts. I had chronic fatigue syndrome and fibromyalgia. If there are any aches or pains present when a doctor brands a patient with chronic fatigue syndrome, the diagnosis of fibromyalgia typically becomes its sidekick. Two years of baffling symptoms affecting both my body and my mind had been reduced to a couple of simple, yet essentially unhelpful, diagnoses defined by chronic muscle pain, fatigue, and sleep problems.

Feeling isolated was another part of this complex health equation that I felt called upon to solve. Not only did I not have the female friendships I craved, I also felt cut off from my artistic self. The demands of my aching body had thwarted my love of creative hobbies, like party-planning, home decorating, crafting, and curating stationery designs. But because I like solving equations and finding solutions to any given roadblock (evidenced in my relentless quest for curing for what ailed me), I figured logic had to be the way out of this mysterious sickness debacle. The scientist in me was taking over as my dominant MO. Researching my illness kept my head above water as I continued to fight the drowning pull of the illness itself.

As I embarked on this research into the root causes of my medical mysteries, Dr. Li planted a seed of hope. She suggested a book based on the latest research about the brain entitled *The Brain That Changes Itself: Stories of Personal Triumph from the Frontiers of Brain Science.* The author, Dr. Norman Doidge, explains the new science of neuroplasticity—the brain's ability to rewire itself. It essentially proves that the mind is powerful enough to heal the body. Contrary to decades of scientific theory, neuroplasticity shows that the adult brain is malleable, and like children we can create new neural connections that serve us instead of sicken us.

These ideas were new to me, and I wanted to learn more, so I checked out some books and online courses on neuroplasticity. I soon discovered Canadian psychologist Annie Hopper's video course, Dynamic Neural Retraining System (DNRS). These DVDs opened my mind to the radical fact that *thoughts alone* can change brain structure, and emotions are powerful enough to strengthen these new connections so that the brain remembers the changes and can let go of old, unhelpful ways of thinking.

I got the strong feeling I was on to something life changing and got to work assimilating and practicing the brain rewiring wisdom Hopper imparted. The primary exercise was to repeat a personalized mantra-infused monologue aloud. In addition, the practice involved reliving pleasant life experiences in my mind. I was so focused on these activities that I put my family responsibilities on hold for three nine-hour days in a row to complete the program from home as diligently as I would have in person.

The tools and techniques I learned translated to what seemed to be real changes in the health of my mind and body. I noticed some positive improvements in my mood and greater optimism, even a mild dissipation of daily symptoms. But the effects were ever so slight, and after a few weeks, I could not stick it out any longer. The training felt forced and intangible. Finding the time and private space to implement these techniques was difficult, and I was not comfortable doing the mantra in front of my kids. I was still seeking that magic pill that would cure me completely. So instead of creating space for a new hour-long daily habit, I continued my path of holistic treatments like nutraceutical supplements and more dietary protocols that I hoped could do the work of healing me instead of letting my body heal itself.

Given the perplexing aches I was enduring, I decided to enlist the help of a weekly massage therapist to at least offer a few hours of heavenly relief from this otherwise ever-present stiffness in my body. The hip pain that had led me to one practitioner after another for almost nine months migrated from the right hip to the left one day. Then, after a Pilates class the following week, the hip cramp floated away completely. It was as if the pain was some sort of stuck energy that, when given room to express itself, was able to glide across my pelvis and out of my body entirely. I could not make much sense of it. The only explanation my scientific mind had to go on was my fibromyalgia diagnosis, which essentially blames a malfunctioning brain for amplified pain signals. My research on the disease suggested that the widespread and often migratory pain is out of proportion to the degree of injury (if there is indeed any muscle injury at all).

One of the drawbacks of being given diagnostic labels for my illnesses was that it was easy to become those labels, to transform those labels into an identity. A few doctors had given me a fibromyalgia label mainly for insurance documentation purposes, but I fortunately had not gotten attached to it. However, my history with insomnia and recent challenges with ever-present exhaustion had over time led to a new self-identity. The Energizer Bunny I had felt myself to be in my twenties was nowhere to be found. I realized that my identity was becoming intricately linked to my fatigue, otherwise known as illness identity. The fear of not sleeping that developed when my son was an infant *had* thwarted my intense efforts to nod off into peaceful oblivion, and now my constant thoughts about how to function in life with my ever-present weariness was fueling the fatigue itself. It was as though my body was self-identifying: *I am Carrie. I am tired.*

Though I had given up a bit prematurely on the DNRS daily practice, many of the concepts I had learned stuck with me. First, I was beginning to understand that letting go of identities like fatigue and pain can be scary once they had established themselves as a part of me. According to the mind-body science I was investigating, we have a primal fear of the unknown, even if the unknown includes an improved level of health. I was beginning to see there were a lot of complicated emotions wrapped up in my dis-ease.

As I was learning to grasp this concept of over-identifying with illness, I came across a quote on social media that pushed me to understand it more. The Buddhist monk and activist Thich Nhat Hanh said, "People have a hard time letting go of their suffering. Out of a fear of the unknown, they prefer suffering that is familiar."

While this quote can be interpreted in many ways, I found it especially relevant to the comfort I received from being sick. I understood sickness. I knew the suffering I was facing every day. I did not give myself the space to contemplate the idea of being well and all that it would mean for me at that point because some deeper part of me feared what that might look like in my day-to-day life. Still not quite ready to let go of my emotional attachment to my illnesses, I continued looking for external solutions to my chronic fatigue and perplexing autoimmune symptoms.

Next up was holistic healthcare. As I continued to need daily naps and suffered from troubling brain fog, I began with a foray into the world of Eastern medicine, including acupuncture, herbal medicine, various forms of massage, and a few other modalities not widely recognized in our Western medical world. There were some dead ends along the way, but in retrospect, all had lessons at their core.

Acupuncture seemed to be as good a place as any to start. My Doctor of Oriental Medicine, Dr. Sara Hartley, is an American-born woman close to my age who had found her way into this work after years trying to find answers to her own health challenges. Acupuncture had been the antidote to her chronic pain, a cure so life altering that it precipitated a career in this field.

Each session began with a check of my pulses (typically weak) and tongue (commonly qi deficient) and intimate questioning about my bowel movements (erratic). Once those were addressed and we had discussed any other nota-ble changes since last time, I expressed my overall despair.

"I still feel exhausted every day. My body is tight, diges-tion is a complete mess, life feels so damn hard. Why am I not getting better?" I asked at one appointment about three months into my treatments.

She looked up from jotting down the latest symptoms in my expanding chart. In her peaceful and understand-ing way, she reminded me that I had been sick for many years, and the body would need at least half that amount of time in which to heal itself. It was not the answer I was looking for, but I guess it was all the reassurance I could expect to get. Healing from the inside out does not come standard with a six-month guarantee. Even if her answer was accurate, I did not know how long I had truly been sick. Had it begun with the respiratory virus that propelled me into chronic daily fatigue, or had my many illnesses been brewing for years (or decades)? I decided to go with the most noticeable shift in my health that had come on the heels of the respiratory virus two years ago. The one that had thwarted my spring break plans and left me sleeping twelve to sixteen hours most days since. *OK, I'm six months into this now, I should be healed in six more months,* I thought with all the optimism I could summon.

I lay down on the acupuncture table, pulled the crisp white sheet up over my chest, and waited for her to gently apply needles to the places that needed it that day— behind my ears, wrists, forehead, toes. I allowed the soft spring breeze to caress my cheeks and then nodded off to the sounds of the tinkling of the wind chimes outside her open window.

A year of biweekly sessions amounted to very little in terms of symptom relief, and although I felt only subtle differences from that modality, I gained a newfound respect for the wisdom of the ancient tradition. Like my functional medicine doctor, Dr. Li, my Doctor of Oriental Medicine took the time to do more than order lab work, ask about symptoms, and send me on my way with a prescription. My new medical team seemed to care about the terrain of my body as a whole. They understood that one organ dances with another; that the texture of my tongue can be a sign of a deficiency in an organ at the other end of my body; that the health of my digestion is vital to the health of every other part of me. This dance taking place inside my body is complex and had become clunky as so many internal and external obstacles had gotten in the way. In order to bring grace and beauty to the dance of my body again I would need help removing those obstacles. I didn't have the patience to wait for this modality to gently bring homeostasis back to my organs, so with haste I moved on to the next thing.

I then tried light touch energy massage and although this, too, did not give me the relief I sought, it introduced me to the concept of the empathic practitioner. Feeling the symptomatic manifestations of another's dis-ease is actually a thing. I witnessed my energy healer wince in pain at the touch of my clenched belly. I was numb to the distress there, but she was not.

Rolfing, a myofascial bodywork system, also seemed

to be a bit of a financial gamble. The intense body-manipulating maneuvers I endured under the hands of a world-renowned practitioner were excruciating. But one bizarre moment of fantastic energy release—which felt like I had wet my pants but thankfully I had not—was possibly the outpouring of my childhood stage-wetting trauma. This practitioner, who had spent half his time working up north with the New York City ballet, also told me on several occasions that I have the graceful essence of a dancer, a seeming paradox to my leopardess, and this comment stuck with me as I continued my healing journey.

Not long after that body manipulating experiment, I began working with an intuitive spiritual guide who told me during one visit that my deceased grandfather had an important message for me.

"Embrace your grace, Care Bear," she said, using the nickname my grandfather had lovingly called me as a child (unbeknownst to my spiritual guide). "Embrace your grace."

I was incredulous at the specificity of this message, yet it started to make sense. To heal, I might need to thank my inner leopardess for her service and begin to unpack the long-hidden vulnerable side of myself, which had been packed away for, well, as long as I could remember. This yin and yang duality correlated to a concept in Chinese medicine I had recently become familiar with—the divine feminine and divine masculine. According to this philosophy, you can be female and display more traditionally masculine qualities, which had been my default approach to life so far. I was used to making the most of my excess energy to move mountains. In the past, I could save the day by taking full advantage of my rational mind and fierce ambition. Logic and perseverance could get me out of most tough situations. But trying to eke out every last ounce of that hustle mentality now (and continuously berating myself for no longer being the person I had always known myself to be) was exhausting. Embracing my grace, and my divine feminine, meant that I would have to lean into a certain stillness that would give me the space to become more open to my feelings. It meant that I would need to allow myself to be vulnerable. Maybe grace meant being open to accepting love and mercy from others—and myself—even though it felt unnatural to me to receive anything from anyone.

The graceful dancer image stayed with me and became a stretch goal. I was unsure of how to embark on this path to my femininity exactly so I circled back to a more logical route. Since food-as-medicine seemed to be something tangible with real benefits (even if their effects had plateaued recently), I enrolled in nutrition classes with the goal of getting my master's degree. Though dietary changes had not quite cured me, nutrition guidance could undoubtedly help others. The majority of individuals in this country are overseen by a broken healthcare system that rewards poor lifestyle choices with Band-Aids paid for by insurance companies. If I am honest, a master's in nutrition and integrative health also sounded prestigious and fed my ego, but it equipped me with the motivation I needed to see this healing process through to the end. This academic path felt rational to me. Once I completed my degree and felt better myself, I reasoned, I could give back to others.

◎ ◎ ◎

Shortly after enrolling in my first round of chemistry and physiology classes, a friend encouraged me to join a small group of women who were starting a spiritual awakening book club. Diving into an unfamiliar topic with a group of strangers who would have me share my feelings on some sort of guided ethereal journey felt terrifying. I was suddenly taken back to Sunday school at my childhood church, stuck in a circle of other middle schoolers who would have rather torn out their fingernails than let intensely guarded emotions run free.

At the same time, I seemed to be getting a nudge to embrace this graceful feminine thing from multiple angles. I warily decided to give the book group a shot and for the next nine months spent my free time reading and discussing a book founded in ancient Toltec wisdom with five other spirit-seeking women. Our regular three-hour gatherings became my initiation into this weirdly uncomfortable, non-logical, heart-centered, vulnerable new world. The book took us on a virtual path to illumination using the plazas, temples, and pyramids of Teotihuacán, Mexico as our guide. Our biweekly meetings included meditations, journaling, and symbolic practices, and ever so slowly began to chisel away at the cement wall I had built around my heart. There was nothing like writing my own obituary (one example of a symbolic practice) to help me see my entire life from an enlightened perspective and rethink how I wanted to spend the rest of my days! The experience taught me that, with a certain willingness to surrender, I could shed the identification with my body, my dis-ease, and even my long-held beliefs. I just had to be willing to trust the unknown.

Though I was not ready to completely give up the known (a concept that was still difficult for my logical mind to grasp) at the end of this nine-month adventure, I had become immersed in a world that forced me to accept the soft friendship of feminine companions. I got the sense I was discovering that beyond my reliance on logic and ambition may lie patience and wisdom, intuition, and, perhaps eventually, healing.

CHAPTER 9

Insidious Mold

BEFORE I COULD STOP MYSELF, THE PLATE WAS slipping from my hands like a Frisbee launched across the backyard. Except in this case, the object was catapulted across the kitchen.

I'm acting like a lunatic, I thought as I continued to hurl expletives—and dishes—across the room. Stunned silent, Matt stood there waiting for the storm to pass. Finally, he walked out the back door, slamming it on the way out. The reverberations lingered in me like waves of shame.

I did not even know what this or any of our mostly one-sided arguments were about. My mind, and my subsequent behavior, felt like it had been taken over by some alien life force, and the real me was powerless to stop it. I was watching the scenes play out around me, while the rational me sat in a chair watching this strange reality.

Turns out our home was filled with mold, and breathing it in constantly was messing with my brain.

In the fall of 2014, we had purchased and moved into

an eclectic '70s home in Sarasota, Florida. It only took a few weeks before I had begun to sense the mustiness, which had been masked by heavy fragrance when we first toured the place during our house-hunting visits. My son had complained from the beginning of itchy eyes, congestion, and coughing, and I soon found myself even more exhausted than my recent norm. Overwhelming bouts of anger seemed to explode out of nowhere, like land mines throughout my world of fatigue and irritability.

We found the first sign of mold two weeks into living in our new home. I had spent the night in my son's room attempting to get a restful night of sleep away from my husband's snoring. I awoke feeling like I had been hit by a train. My head was cloudy and congested, my face was swollen and distorted, and I felt like I could barely see straight. I had attributed my son's cold-like symptoms to a virus. Now the more likely cause seemed like an amplified allergic reaction.

Perhaps it was the list of renovations the sellers told us they had completed over the years and the all-clear we got from our home inspection and additional mold inspection before we closed, but somehow I had been placated into thinking nothing was amiss. Now I began to suspect mold. I smelled the mustiness that filled my olfactory receptors. It was in there, in my son's room, and he'd been exposed all night, every night since day one.

I tracked down a few indoor air quality technicians, and the clean-up began with a thorough scrubbing of the AC ducts. When that was not enough to quell the odor, our particularly thorough mold inspector followed the clues to a leaky attic air handler that had left black mold colonies beneath the paint on my son's walls. Then we uncovered rotten wood framing in a closet that had previously been a bathroom. It would be almost a year before the mold removal process culminated in removing all the upstairs flooring and door frames and stripping half the house down to the studs. It was as if a water bomb had gone off years before in my son's centrally located bedroom. With the help of the humid Florida air, the mold spores had been replicating ever since in a twelve-foot radius.

Here we were about nine months after having moved into this cesspool of hidden fungal growth and my anger was back, more unpredictable than ever. In the wake of my latest fit of uncontrolled rage, my family scattered in all directions. I was left to pick up the pieces, literally and metaphorically. I swept up the shards of broken plate so that Pippin, our new Brittany spaniel and the only one brave enough to stay behind with me in this otherwise abandoned kitchen, would not nick a paw. Then I slid into my flip flops and quietly slipped out the front door, head hanging low.

I smelled the new sprouts of baby jasmine reaching up along the mailbox post. I began to walk west toward the grand houses enhanced with sea grapes, saw palmettos, and beautyberries overlooking the serene Sarasota Bay. Taking solo walks along the lush, charmingly quaint streets near our home never failed to bring a sense of calm to a body often wound tighter than spandex on an elephant.

During several of our appointments, Dr. Li had stressed to me the importance of spending time in nature. She explained that the simple act of walking outside and connecting to the earth through all our senses—tuning in to the textures, tastes, sights, and smells of the world around us—bridges the gap between our overthinking minds and our intuitive physical bodies. The smell of a tree, naturally suffused with health-giving compounds, has been proven to elicit a calming response from head to toe. This deliciously soft interlude between intense segments of the drama playing out in our home was exactly what we all needed.

The peace I managed to find on those walks was unfortunately short-lived, as my sense of smell was advancing at lightning speed. Navigating the outside world was increasingly challenging. I quickly switched off the air conditioning in the car whenever a whiff of exhaust came through the vents to prevent the inhalation of and subsequent headache from the toxic gas. I often cut my neighborhood walks short if I passed the home of someone drying their clothes, as detecting the chemically-laden dryer sheets in the air made me dizzy. My turbocharged sense of smell became so debilitating it challenged my sense of sanity. It was like I had the nose of a bloodhound but still could not sniff out the trail to healing.

The mud-in-my-veins fatigue wouldn't let up and my head always felt cloudy. I was determined to get us out of this mess, and I started with online research into this insidious toxin. I had to find out how the mold could be affecting my health.

I recalled a fellow mystery illness sufferer in an online support group I frequented having mentioned a film called *Moldy* a few months back. This seemed like as good a time as any to make the relatively small investment in the DVD. The documentary, the brainchild of Dave Asprey, founder and CEO of Bulletproof and creator of the popular Bulletproof Coffee, features many of the country's top medical experts along with several mold illness survivors. As I watched I became absorbed in the stories of others who had once faced similar symptoms to the ones I was experiencing. Following their accounts brought a sense of relief, despair, and hope all at the same time. Relief that my health had not gotten so bad I was forced to live in a tent in the desert as one victim had. Despair that something as ubiquitous as mold could wreak such havoc on a person's body. Hope that there might finally be a clear therapeutic opportunity available to me.

Mold illness, or chronic inflammatory response syndrome (CIRS), is a condition defined by a collection of symptoms and often results from exposure to mold in water-damaged buildings. Dr. Ritchie Shoemaker, the main physician highlighted in the movie, developed a protocol based on his decades of research into this illness. Given all that we had been going through with the house, I had to pursue this further. I wanted to find out just how much mold was playing a part in my body's bizarre collapse, so I located a physician trained in Shoemaker's particular diagnostic and treatment methods.

Meanwhile, Dr. Li was continuing to help me manage my MTHFR, a trend in the functional medical community and one that she was well versed in. The acronym does not stand for motherf*@%er, as many friends joked when I tried to explain my homozygous A1298C gene mutation to pairs of bewildered eyes. No, it stands for methylenete-trahydrofolate reductase, the name for both the gene and the resulting enzyme that stimulates crucial biochemical reactions in your body, namely a process called methylation. This biochemical process, which has a significant impact on the regulation of many organ systems, includes the transfer of one carbon atom and three hydrogen atoms from one place to another. My chemistry knowledge was a bit rusty at this point, but I got the idea.

Under her care, I was gently introducing supplements like folate (the active form of folic acid) and a specific type of vitamin B12 to my daily regimen to help the detoxification process of a body that was struggling to properly rid itself of an overabundance of chemicals, heavy metals, and other inflammatory offenders. While this gentle process may have been working, I eventually got impatient and began to navigate the management of my diagnosis outside the confines of my functional medicine physician.

I had now been presented with diagnoses for a few genetic wild cards—confirmed MTHFR and suspected CIRS. Impairment by these hereditary traits seemed disheartening, yet I realized they are both quite common. I read estimates indicating that as much as fifty percent of some ethnicities have at least one MTHFR variant and twenty-four percent of the population is mold susceptible.

Wanting to know more, I returned to Bruce Lipton's *The Biology of Belief,* which I had explored with my book group a year and a half earlier. The major takeaway I got from Lipton's work was that genes are not the solo players in our inherited fate; instead, we can control our destiny.

This is the main idea behind the term epigenetics, a concept that figures largely in Lipton's work. As I understand it, epigenetics gained traction in the 1990s, and a plethora of groundbreaking studies entered the scene in the early 2000s. In one of these studies, researchers found that genetic "hitchhikers" can modify DNA and control genetic expression.

From what I gathered, the MTHFR gene and other genetic variations commonly found between genes in the DNA lead to a decreased ability to detoxify. Mercury is a good example. Having these genetic variations can inhibit the body's ability to excrete a portion of ingested or absorbed mercury. I certainly did not need an explanation for how mercury and other heavy metals can ravage the body. Exposure in utero and in early childhood development is of particular concern because mercury is toxic to the brain, kidneys, and immune system.

Where I grew up playing with mercury was a well-known pastime. Breaking open the thermometer and feeling the deliciously cold slippery metal ball in my hand had not been a cause for concern. Neither were the metal fillings that topped off the cavities in my baby teeth. Thank goodness I never had any in my permanent chops, but many other people are unknowingly walking around with mouths full of mercury.

Other gene hitchhikers wreaking havoc on epigenetic processes include many toxins like heavy metals (beyond mercury), pesticides, polycyclic aromatic hydrocarbons (found in vehicle exhaust, tobacco smoke, and grilled meats), synthetic hormones, radiation, viruses, and bacteria. I was realizing that those insidious environmental toxins went beyond just disrupting my endocrine system, as I had discovered after my previous lackluster encounters with the two endocrinologists. These epigenetic changes have also been linked to a wide range of chronic health conditions, including autoimmunity, Alzheimer's disease, birth defects, and cancer. Even worse, these increasingly prevalent environmental toxins, to which I had been exposed most of my life, can actually alter DNA.

What I learned from Bruce Lipton and other epigenetic researchers was that my genetic destiny, which was once thought to be fixed at birth, can be influenced both negatively and positively by lifestyle and environment. The combination of a growing number of toxins in our homes, our environments, and our food, along with deep-seated emotional wounds and life stressors, can spell a recipe for mystery illness disaster, much of which can be traced to detrimental mutated genes. However, I found comfort in the understanding that pernicious gene expression can be reversed.

According to experts, the antidote to these harmful hitchhikers can be found in beneficial lifestyle measures like a healthful diet, the right nutritional supplements, meditation or prayer, communing with nature, connecting with others, exercise, rest, play, and finding your life purpose or passions.

I would soon learn that many of these non-nutritional antidotes were doable as long as I was willing to let my body lead the way. They required creating a few new habits—like making space for a short guided meditation and morning walk every day—and rediscovering many of life's simple pleasures in ways that I had lost touch with somewhere along the path into adulthood. Connecting to my purpose and my passions was a bit more difficult, but I had the sense that going back to school with the goal of eventually helping others was a step in the right direction.

Diet and supplementation were easy, at least in the sense that I could always lean on my mind to help me tackle these lifestyle modifications. I was still trying to figure out what a healthful diet meant for me. I was often more confused than comforted by the various "Eat and Enjoy" and "Avoid or Limit" lists on the latest trendy diets. I had embarked on an entire year without any form of sugar aside from berries in an attempt to rid myself of the candida I concluded must have been plaguing my gut and brain. I had endured the "keto flu" that came along with the high-fat, minimal carb diet that purported to help with some autoimmune conditions. Now, with my doctor's guidance, I was attempting to treat myself with yet more dietary protocols with weird names like AIP and low FODMAPs to combat the GI distress that increasingly ailed me. So much for letting go and letting my intuition be my guide. My gut instincts apparently weren't fine-tuned enough at that point, or I didn't have the patience to let the healing process run its course.

My functional medicine doctor had been cautious about labeling my dis-ease, but she did suggest my body was behaving in ways that mimicked autoimmunity. I learned that there are currently over one hundred identified autoimmune conditions. Western medicine defines these as diseases in which a person's immune system attacks his or her own tissue, the very cells it is meant to protect. It seemed to fit, as I was building an arsenal of reasons to believe that my broken body was failing me.

Given this autoimmune state I was potentially in, the ketogenic diet seemed worth a shot. But after a month I wondered if my hormones could be taking a hit, therefore offsetting any benefits. I assumed I was close to perimenopause at this point based on a maternal lineage of early period cessation and an irregular menstrual cycle. My research indicated that during the transition (and in times of stress in general) hormones fluctuate so much that they need carbohydrates to support and balance them. Plus, I missed them. I was not sure if it was an unhealthy craving or a true cellular hunger, but I wanted carbs!

Even though I was just beginning my nutrition degree, it was becoming clear to me that drastically manipulating my diet could have a significant influence on the gut's terrain as well and not necessarily to my benefit. I had recently come across one theory suggesting that opportunistic pathogens thrive when a diet is low in plant foods and high in meat, dairy, and processed food. If this was the case, then my foray into the keto world may have taken down a few strains of bacteria, while providing fuel for other, lesser-known pathogens to thrive. I had done my best to avoid processed food, but meat was a key component of every meal and dairy had made a reappearance in my diet. Another theory proposed that by withholding carbs, our beneficial bacteria may feed on the lining of our guts, leading right back to leaky gut.

At the very least, I understood the basics of fresh, nutrient-dense food. Sourcing local, pesticide-free produce and free-range, grass-fed meat, and shopping the perimeter of the grocery store instead of the center aisles were the closest I could get to eating the way Mother Nature intended.

◎ ◎ ◎

A few months later I was sitting face-to-Skype with Dr. Miles Gregory, a board-certified internist who had transformed his practice into one of the few in the country helping CIRS patients. After we had discussed ad nauseam my ongoing list of symptoms—a list that now also included an extremely narrow window of temperature tolerance and the need to urinate every hour during the day and several times at night—he asked what medications I was currently taking.

"Oh, just low dose naltrexone," I responded, with the assumption that he would know exactly what I was talking about. It was 2015, and although this treatment approach had been recognized for its anti-inflammatory and immune-modulating effects since the 1980s, it had only recently begun gaining momentum as a standard treatment. At this point, its off-label use (less than one tenth the standard dose) was generally restricted to alternative practitioners.

"I'm sorry?" he offered his ear into the Skype camera as if he had misheard me. I repeated it clearly, which seemed to confuse him more. Naltrexone, at doses starting at 50 mg per day, is FDA-approved for the treatment of alcohol and opiate abuse.

He scribbled some notes and cautiously asked, "Are you on . . . narcotics? Or is it for pain?"

"No, low dose naltrexone is . . . No, um . . . Do you know about low dose naltrexone?" This was bizarre. It looked like I may have to try to talk medical jargon to a medical doctor. I was not sure I was qualified.

"I know about it from a chronic pain standpoint," he offered, no hint of superiority or judgment in his voice whatsoever. I loved this man. A curious and receptive doctor. How had I gotten so lucky?

"Okay, well, my functional medicine doctor recommended it to help get my immune system calm and to help with gut stuff. There's a good bit of research on the subject right now. It seems to be helping."

"Okay." He did not have much to contribute to this. He moved on. "What supplements are you taking?"

As I attempted to explain the liver support supplement the newly appointed nutraceutical pharmacist in me had recently added to my repertoire, I noticed the expression draining from his face. "It has something called biopterin because apparently, people with A1298C homozygous MTHFR have trouble converting phenylalanine to tyrosine. So I started taking this because it has the biopterin I need to convert those, along with dandelion root, milk thistle, broccoli extract, green tea, and NADH. I'm taking less than one tenth of a capsule per day because I'm so sensitive." Hearing myself talk, I realized I was also a bit insane attempting to self-supplement like this. What the hell was I doing?

I noticed a slight nod and a "hmmm" from him, but his face was now completely blank. Not surprising since allopathic doctors did not generally keep up with the ever-expanding, loosely regulated world of vitamins and herbs. My list of supplements continued: a multivitamin with methyl folate and B12, magnesium, L-theanine, vitamins D3 and K2, spore-based probiotic, and iodoral (self-prescribed nano-dose again).

He continued his new patient interview by asking about family health history and my past careers, which somehow led to a discussion about my self-induced pressure to achieve perfection. Dr. Gregory seemed to have already picked up on this (perhaps from my lengthy discourse on supplements) and offered some spiritual wisdom about competition and the misconception that lack even exists, especially important information for us card-carrying type A members. His compassionate demeanor put me at ease.

We then segued into a discussion about CIRS and my potential encounters with water-damaged buildings in childhood, school, jobs, and currently (and most obviously) in our nine-month home remediation project. Then we moved on to the results of my pre-appointment, ridiculously expensive slew of blood analyses.

"One out of four people in the US have a genetic predisposition to CIRS. Those of you with it don't recognize certain chemicals in your environment as being foreign to your body. One of the functions of your vast immune system is to look at every particle that goes through your bloodstream and recognize if it's 'Carrie' (self) or whether it's foreign." The light in his face was back on, and his hands were moving animatedly. He was in full-on teaching mode. I nodded so he would continue.

He went on to explain that a built-in sensory system will tag the foreign particles so that my immune system will know to ramp up and attack them. I broke our eye contact and began writing in my notebook (a few key words and a bit of doodling, actually) to appear studious.

"This adaptive immune system is one of the things that protects us from infections from bacteria mold, viruses, and some chemicals." Yes, I was aware of the complexity of the immune system. His simplified explanation made sense to me. He continued, "But one out of four people has this genetic predisposition, and you don't recognize certain pathogens and chemicals as being foreign when they get inside your body. You make no effort to get rid of them. They just accumulate. Over time, these toxins find different ways to trigger your immune system until eventually, your immune system becomes triggered all the time."

He also explained that our knowledge of the science is always catching up and the latest understanding is that the recognized foreign bodies are not being presented properly for the formation of antibodies in those of us with CIRS. Pathogens and chemicals get tagged, but the immune system does not adequately take care of them. Either way, my immune system was on the fritz and leaving my body in a state of chronic inflammation.

Good news: I had a new treatment path that included various medications to help rid my body of the built-up toxic load that was weighing me down. While I felt relief in having what felt like a legitimate diagnosis for the first time, my outlook was clouded by my past experiences with treatment paths that fell short. Previous diagnoses of chronic fatigue, fibromyalgia, mood swings as part of the package of being a mom, and some fancy new MTHFR genetic label hadn't come with solutions, just near-empty words for the medical mystery I had become. I was cautiously optimistic that with this treatment I could feel significantly better in the next six to nine months.

Bad news: Dr. Gregory explained to me that based on my lab work and our discussion of my symptoms I had a lifelong illness—not just CIRS, but the dreaded multi-susceptible human leukocyte antigens (HLA) gene. This most problematic of the genetic deviations of HLA, which helps the immune system differentiate between body tissue and foreign substances, apparently leaves me vulnerable to relapses when exposed to a number of possible toxins. I had tested positive for eight of the ten physiological or genetic markers for this newly discovered disease state. Diagnosis was confirmed with just five.

He told me that I would need to avoid water-damaged moldy buildings for the rest of my life. In addition to mold, pathogens that could trigger and complicate my chronic inflammatory response included Lyme spirochetes and various toxins found in fish and algae. The majority of those run rampant in Florida, where I lived. To add insult to injury, he explained that additional medication would be required to manage my chemical sensitivities forever.

CIRS became my latest identity as days revolved around researching how my body was defective and why I was dealt this genetic pair of deuces while so many others were holding a hand that allowed them more frequent wins. I guess it was a good thing I had chemical sensitivities and could smell danger like a well-trained drug detection dog. But this mold-avoidance sentence was nearly impossible to adhere to when the experts interviewed in *Moldy* estimated that more than half of homes in the US had some degree of fungal growth. To make matters worse, we had made a life in humid Florida, where upwards of ninety percent of buildings are likely to be affected.

CHAPTER 10

Fight or Flight

SHORTLY AFTER BEING GIVEN THESE NEW DIAG-noses, a notification showed up in my Facebook feed for Annie Hopper's DNRS workshop tailored toward people suffering from chronic fatigue, fibromyalgia, multiple chemical sensitivities, and . . . yep, mold illness. The harmony of it all was that the event, which usually took place in the western US or in Canada, the creator's home country, would take place in Florida the following month.

This was an in-person version of the DVD program that I had briefly delved into a few years earlier when I had begun working with my functional medicine doctor.

At the time, I had not been fully open to putting the techniques into a dedicated practice, mostly because the premise required engaging in inner work that did not come naturally to me. I just wasn't good at it; I pre-ferred researching and implementing a diet or a pill that could make all the problems go away. I gravitated to hard science and research over playing around with emotions and focusing my attention within.

But the fact that this in-person event showed up basically down the road could not make the path being laid out for me any more apparent. At the same time, the emerging topic of neuroplasticity had gained momentum since I had last dabbled in it, and the argument that the brain has an innate ability to change itself in ways that could lead to real physical healing in the body had gained traction in the medical world. The idea that maybe I would not have to succumb to a lifelong attachment to medications was potentially life-changing, and I felt I needed to take a second look at this ground-breaking practice.

So I traveled to Bonita Springs, Florida, where I met nineteen other people suffering from mystery illnesses just like me. Through a series of video presentations, lectures, and breakout sessions, we first learned how the body can get out of whack to begin with.

I had heard this analogy before: A caveman is chased by a predator (such as a tiger) and either defends himself or runs for dear life. In this scenario, his flight-or-flight response has kicked in. Adrenaline and cortisol flood the bloodstream. His heart rate and blood pressure rise, pupils dilate, and airways open. Blood is diverted to big muscles needed for running and jumping at the expense of small muscles like the ones that keep your bladder tight. (So wetting one's pants becomes a possibility. Hmm . . . memories of a particular math bee mishap come to mind.)

His amygdala, the brain's fear center, sends nerve cells to the prefrontal cortex, the part of the brain responsible for judgment and reasoning, to quiet it. Amid this threat to his life, the last thing he has time to do is rationalize his response. His primal urges are more critical than impulse control in this situation.

I was reminded that this scenario is what our sympathetic nervous system is meant to do to protect us from being attacked by a wild animal. But once the threat is over the parasympathetic nervous system, the "rest-and-digest" response, steps back in, and the caveman is able to sit around the campfire with ease—laughing, singing, and dancing. The thing was, I soon realized, I was not doing a whole lot of laughing, singing, or dancing these days. If I were to be honest, I did not feel the inclination to engage in any sort of play. My body felt like it was in a chronic state of tension and was either amped up or completely knocked out. The caveman analogy could not be more relevant.

We also learned that a body stuck in a chronic state of fight-or-flight has an immune system which functions erroneously and sometimes can have a lack of impulse control; or in my case, it had ongoing bodily inflammation and a whopping dose of crazy. This all seemed to tie in to my recent CIRS diagnosis. My immune system was apparently facing an uphill battle having been heavily taxed by various environmental triggers on top of a genetic predisposition for dysfunction.

The facilitators of our program put a lot of emphasis on the limbic system, the part of the brain that influences the autonomic nervous system (i.e. sympathetic and parasympathetic branches). They explained that from an evolutionary perspective, the limbic system is said to be one of the most primitive parts of the brain. One very important way that the limbic system impacts health is by carrying sensory input from the environment to the hypothalamus—the small brain region producing hormones that control things like body temperature, hunger, and mood—and then from the hypothalamus to other parts of the body. The hypothalamus acts like the regulator of hormone control, helps the body maintain balance, and sends signals to the pituitary, thyroid, and adrenal glands. The limbic system receives information from many body parts, including the heart, vagus nerve, digestive system, and skin. Because of the hypothalamus's functions, the limbic system is directly in control of your stress response (fight-or-flight).

Here is where it got even more interesting. In many individuals with mystery illness, we learned, accumulation of traumas to the brain—infections, chemical exposure, physical injury, emotional distress, and genetic predispositions—all activate the stress response. An over-activated stress response ultimately leads to abnormal sensory perception, which sets off a protective process as if, like the caveman running from the tiger, your very life depended on it. Over time, this hypervigilance results in a heightened reaction to even a relatively minor exposure to triggers.

As I returned to my room at the recently refurbished Shangri-La hotel and spa that first night, I found that I had more to contend with than simply digesting this wealth of information from the seminar. While the facility had taken great pains to be sure that only fragrance-free, non-toxic cleaning products and linens had been used in our rooms, we were told, they apparently were not able to address a very apparent mold problem. Having been through our year of hell, I was likely more qualified than anyone there to detect, investigate, and conduct the orchestra of specialists who would have been needed to clean it up. *Just because they didn't see it didn't mean it wasn't there,* I thought. Not wanting to make a fuss, I put off approaching the staff.

I pried open my painted-in, rust-jammed windows to let in some air. The humid air would only fuel any existing mold, I realized, so it was a no-win situation. But I did not know what else to do, so I left the window open for an hour or so until I heard what was likely the groundskeeper's truck driving around the property. I shut the windows again to block out the vehicle's ear-piercing back-up beeper, and I continued my fitful night of very little sleep.

I could see what was going on from a new perspective now, given all that I was learning at this program and recalling what I had read in Norman Doidge's work about neuroplasticity. My hyperactive limbic system was dealing with a mix of my conscious fear of and actual exposure to the fungi that had wounded me many times before. When the brain tries for too long to help you, by adapting to compensate for injury and disease, it can get stuck in fight-or-flight mode. This acute adjustment in response to new situations or changes in the environment ends up being a chronic adjustment as the limbic system becomes maladapted. While I understood that the amount of mold in this hotel room may or may not have been detrimental to my health (because now with my heightened sense of smell I could detect environmental toxins at relatively low levels), my brain was telling my body that it certainly was. But knowing this was not enough to change my body's response, so after waking up achy and inflamed, I chose to drive the two hours home to sleep and return early each day for the remainder of the program, grateful that I lived close enough to do so.

The next few days we dove further into the science of the nervous system as it related to our shared mystery illnesses. Apparently, current research suggests that as the brain learns to issue a constant stream of alert chemical/hormone messages to inform the rest of the body that there is a problem, many critical body functions—digestion, hormone production, tissue repair—are put on the back burner, so to speak.

We also examined the distinction between the fight-or-flight and the rest-and-repair (or rest-and-digest) response. When our body learns to default to the parasympathetic nervous system (rest-and-repair), it is much better able to do what it is designed to do: heal. The immune system balances out, the GI tract starts running smoothly again, and the rest of the organ systems return to doing the work for which they are made.

Once we understood that our bodies were stuck in fight-or-flight, we began to learn methods and techniques that would help us mobilize our minds to direct our limbic systems. The biggest ah-ha moment for me in this portion of the training was that thoughts *alone* have the potential to change brain structure. This was not as simplistic as "mind over matter" or "it's all in your head," as I heard some skeptics say over the years. When the body is stuck in a "limbic system trauma loop," as Annie Hopper, the program's director calls it, we are constantly consumed by our physical, psychological, and emotional manifestations and the triggers outside of us that perpetuate our dis-ease. Our primal limbic brain is dedicated to protecting us (on an unconscious level) so it takes deliberate conscious effort for us to go inward and become aware of the repetitive thoughts, feelings, and behaviors that need to be interrupted in order to break the loop. With the facilitator's guidance we investigated our individual core beliefs and learned to become curious observers of our repetitive thoughts and feelings. We learned that awareness was the first step to breaking these chronic patterns so that established neural connections in the brain could begin to be severed and eventually rewired in ways that heal instead of sicken.

After a few days of digging into the thoughts, feelings, and experiences that were governing our limbic system dysfunction (our trauma loops) through various introspective journaling activities and small group discussions, we learned the practical neural retraining steps. These steps included a mix of physical movements (proven to add oomph to the rewiring process), a monologue (designed to break patterns, re-label symptoms, and affirm a new mental path forward), and visualizations (enhanced by enlisting our five senses). I finally got comfortable repeating my own custom affirmation despite the initial awkwardness of declaring it out loud to a room full of participants. "I am filled with grace, gratitude, and love of life," I proclaimed, while opening my arms wide like I was receiving the message. Eventually, over the course of the week, these steps became second nature to me.

The greatest benefit of the week was learning to freely access my sense of joy, an expansive, tear-inducing high that had long since gone dormant. We had learned to develop a library of three to four visualizations based on pleasant memories that we could call upon when needed. For me, the memory of my first son's birth as he was gently placed on my breast filled me with immense joy and wonder; I recalled a euphoric moment from my wedding as I walked across the lush church lawn to the sanctuary while my best friend held the train of my dress behind me. Recalling these sensations, I was learning, sent a cascade of powerful healing hormones and chemicals through my body every time. The more I could access this state, the more I could initiate the parasympathetic nervous system response meant to heal me. With plenty of live rehearsals under our belts, we were set free to continue the daily practice at home.

◎ ◎ ◎

While trying to visualize past scenarios to the point of inner bliss would take months of practice to achieve consistently, when I first felt an explosion of love emanating from my heart again, I knew that I was home. This mostly indescribable sensation feels like colorful threads of intense joy, sadness, longing, hope, gratitude, and safety all tied together in a beautifully crafted bow. At least that is the best I can concoct in words to describe this inner awakening. It happened infrequently at first.

But, with repeated work (because as ironic as it sounds, creating blissful visualizations is work for those of us who have become so disconnected from the experience), I fell steadily into that space within me. I was also able to recognize and capture these small but magical moments in real time more and more.

Because the progress wasn't constant, I found the exercise to be difficult. It was no easy feat. No magic pill. The practice I carried home with me from my workshop at the Shangri-La required that I dedicate a minimum of one hour each day to engaging my mind and body in that series of specific mental exercises. This discipline was certainly a far cry from the Band-Aid approaches I had applied in my early Western medicine days. No, this mind-body "work" to investigate my inner emotional world required dedication, effort, and blind faith to a degree that I had not experienced before.

I was now able to recognize that summoning the energy to take a walk around the neighborhood, join the family in a spirited game of backyard baseball, or make it to the neighborhood yoga class would pay off in the end with a boost in mood and mental clarity. The hourlong daily process of getting here, though, was so fundamentally different than the outside-in modalities I had explored. Using my psyche as my starting point was novel territory and so much more laborious than all I had tried thus far.

It felt like there was a constant inner battle going on inside my head: Why did I always seem to have to either overcome fatigue or succumb to it in order to heal? Why was fatigue this permanent fixture in my life that had to constantly be addressed (which was really being resisted)? What was it trying to teach me?

It must be here to impart some sort of life lesson. Why else is it sticking around? the budding spiritual seeker in me thought.

I was truly feeling better in many ways. My mind was clearer; I was finding joy again; I knew how to reframe my symptoms (even some of my friends had come to request the services of my super sniffer). I looked forward to my days. But the resentment I felt about my body's lingering weaknesses, namely less-than-robust energy, continued to gnaw at my psyche. The mental and emotional energy I expended resisting, judging, critiquing its weariness was exhausting.

While I continued to engage in an inner energy battle, lightbulbs were going on all around me as I incorporated as many of these healthy measures as possible into my life. I was now adjusting to the new routine of a daily neuro-plasticity practice, and I found myself overcome by the desire to keep the feel-good hormones of the visualization practices alive as much as I could. I realized that *living* what I was visualizing (laughing, playing, being in nature) was an effective way to feel good. Imagine that! Sometimes I would find the rigid determination to make sure I was feeding myself and my family conscientiously at odds with my longing for the ease of letting go and enjoying the simplicity of life.

Here is the analogy I came up with to help me understand the level of work and commitment required: It is like a second baseman who dreams of pitching. He would never be moved from his regular position on a base to the pitcher's mound in the middle of a big game without having done hours of drills and training. His arm and wrist would not know how to interact with his mind optimally to pull off skilled pitches, especially under pressure. The disciplined practices done outside of the intensity of the game prepare his mind and body for success in the heat of the moment.

The same is true with the brain rewiring steps I learned at the DNRS workshop. Dedicating ample time every day (when not symptomatic or triggered by environmental stressors) would eventually create new neural pathways in my brain necessary for the successful rerouting of my otherwise automatic and overactive stress response. Self-directed neuroplasticity would soon turn out to be my biggest ticket to health freedom.

Another part of this process that felt doable to me right away was the idea of reframing my illness. I became adept at noticing that my old stories to go along with symptoms carried messages of powerlessness, despair, body obsession, avoidance measures, and isolation. I needed new stories, or the old ones would always take me down.

I decided to start the reframing process with my abnormally heightened sense of smell. Much like a canary in a coal mine, many of us with mystery illnesses have an exceptional ability to detect harmful toxins before those around us do. Mold was not the only environmental toxin I was adept at sniffing out. The plethora of fragrances at places like Bed Bath & Beyond were beyond avoidable once you got into the store. While at one time, strolling the aisles of kitchen gadgets and high thread count sheets had felt like a luxury, I now kept myself away from those types of stores. Paint fumes, chemical air fresheners, engine exhaust, perfumes, new car interiors, furniture upholstery, cigarette smoke, road construction tar . . . I could smell it all, amplified.

I wanted to try and discover how this symptom could be comingled with certain fear-based emotions or repetitive mind chatter. Whenever an intense smell overwhelmed me, I took a moment to stop and breathe. I noted some anxiety, like a lurching in my chest and weakness in my legs, when I detected an environmental toxin. The immediate trepidation I felt as I got a whiff of mold, dryer exhaust, or vehicle emissions, I believe, played a large part in my subsequent headaches. I knew that those toxins were bad for me; therefore, my limbic brain would go into hypervigilant mode. I was beginning to understand that this state of fight-or-flight, when switched on too hastily and too often, could lead to dis-ease in the body. Knowledge is power, as they say, and recognizing this connection was a big step toward reframing this symptom.

I had two young boys who were obsessed with DC and Marvel movies, and I had grown to love them myself. I learned to think of my ability to perceive danger through my sense of smell as my superpower. Several friends and family members had even requested the assistance of my nose to vet their homes and businesses for mold, and I was happy to oblige as long as I didn't have to stick around for long if I detected the all too familiar musty stench.

CHAPTER 11

It's (Not) All Good

WITH MY INNER LEOPARDESS BURIED INSIDE, I prided myself on being agreeable and avoiding confrontation. Shaping my persona to best harmonize with whomever I was with got me through life. On the outside, I smiled and nodded in agreement even when I disagreed on the inside. Speaking my truth felt too risky, especially in school and social circles. But through my new mindfulness work, I began to see that my inside often didn't match my outside. I was not being true to myself, my needs, or my feelings. I was not being authentic.

I stopped listening to my intuition early in life. I remember my high school boyfriend, Jason, kept me at a distance except when convenient for him, and I never broke free from the role of the innocent conciliatory girlfriend. He taunted me over the phone with hints of infidelity that I politely shrugged off. He never introduced me to his friends when I drove up to see him at his college. All decisions were dictated by him, with little to no input on my part. But his sharp wit could light up a room. At least, that was the view through my lens. I assumed everyone was as mesmerized by him as I was.

I almost do not blame him. My lack of backbone had to have been palpable. Not only did it trap me in some weak shell, but it probably made me less desirable to him. It is no wonder he ultimately broke up with me on my front porch steps on the way out the door of another isolated weekend together. At least he was gentleman enough to do so in person.

I continued living outside my integrity well beyond high school, as evidenced by the way I handled my phar-maceutical sales career in my twenties. The dog and pony show I had felt obliged to put on as part of my job (the fancy lunches and showy gifts, the feigned interest in the office manager's kids, the exaggerated smile painted onto my face seconds before walking in the door) had been exhausting. Sure, there were some genuine connections that I honestly enjoyed. There were a few doctors and staff members with whom I shared mutual respect and inter-ests, but many were phony, manufactured relationships based on a transactional exchange.

As I now see it, my body did not begin showing me the ramifications of suppressing my truth and allowing others' behavior to dictate mine until years later. Now that I was working so hard to keep my nervous system in balance, I was more aware than ever of circumstances that could tip the scales in favor of my fight-or-flight tendencies, i.e. increased heart rate, shallow breathing, uncomfortable gut sensations. I have always thought my ability to put people at ease and effortlessly blend in with their personas to be socially beneficial. Having grown up in the South to be a "Southern Belle," I knew all too well the effects of female persuasion. While I still believe amenable communication is important, I have to be careful not to fall into its easy trap. If I focus too much on others and how they feel (or how I think they feel), then I can find myself outside the lines of my integrity pretty quickly.

Confronted with political discussions, child-rearing advice, or religious preferences, my mind will override my body in these situations frequently to appease an uncomfortable situation taking place outside of me. I might let out a slight chuckle or a polite nod of assumed agreement, my mind easily swayed in the direction of my companion. As I was beginning to pay close attention, though, I noticed that my body was often saying otherwise. In those moments, any number of organs could go awry, not just a racing heart or clenching stomach. I have felt everything from a choking sensation to a burning headache in those moments as well.

When both my mind and body are saying "no," and my actions go the opposite direction, I am really living outside my integrity. This scenario most often happens when I find myself entangled with a person of authority, someone intensely opinionated, or a narcissist. Take, for example, the endocrinologist who years before had told me in no uncertain terms (and without the slightest consideration for my opinion) that a pill would fix me. The risk of upsetting the tone of the conversation can outweigh all the nudges of my mind and body. Social constructs keep me locked in my internal discord. In that case, more love for and trust in myself could have kept me from taking the thyroid medication that had made me so wired and angry. Living outside my integrity back then, I did not believe I was worth the confrontation, and at the time I honestly did not know where else to turn to feel better.

I have found that a little bit of tact can get me through uncomfortable encounters without compromising my values. Maybe a neutral nod of the head or simple "hmm" is all that is required in the moment, especially if the other person is a casual acquaintance. Acknowledgment, reflection, and a touch of self-forgiveness afterward tends to release the negative energy that would otherwise have festered inside me. I recalled that by the end of the appointment with the second endocrinologist I had made headway by tossing her script in the wastebasket. The liberation I had experienced was the result of veering closer to my integrity. As I was becoming more aware of the nudges of my physical body, I was slowly getting better at it.

We all have an internal truth meter. Whether or not we choose to tap into it beneath the layers of politeness and trauma we have accumulated is our choice. On several occasions I have caught myself trying to make someone feel better or less awkward after their inappropriate comment as if I could ease their embarrassment, or the embarrassment I assume they must feel. It is highly unlikely that they even noticed their gaffe. Case in point, mustering the courage to let a friend know that I do not agree with his sexist/racist/homophobic comment can end up being just the impetus needed to move us both out of a habitual pattern: mine of ignoring the urge to say what I feel is right for fear of intensifying the discomfort and him the chance to think about how his belief may be pigheaded. His hurtful viewpoint gets disrupted and questioned while the grip of inauthenticity in my body lets up a bit. I have found that the more I speak my truth, no matter how insignificant the situation may seem, the more harmonized my body feels. A body out of harmony can manifest in symptoms of dis-ease.

Looking back, I was faced with this truth before but had failed to see how completely it affected my body and mind. In the summer of 2013 my vegan chef friend, Laura, had asked me to join her on a consult with a client who was having difficulty with raw foods. He wanted to try bone broth, and she was not equipped to provide this level of service. Beef marrow, oxtails, neck bones, chicken feet . . . these were not exactly part of a raw vegan chef's repertoire, and I had become somewhat of a pro in this department as of late. I had had to force myself to drink countless mugs of the stuff as part of the GAPS and Paleo diets I had formerly committed myself to. Once I did a bit of research on the subject, I learned that roasting the bones before adding the other ingredients (vegetables, apple cider vinegar, salt, and water) was key to improving the flavor and aroma.

Being invited along to the appointment with Laura and her client was an exciting twist of fate. I was there not as a patient but as a practitioner of sorts. This scenario was a new role for me, and I attempted to play the part with as much authority and enthusiasm as I could invoke.

As I proceeded to walk my friend, her client, and a few of his family members through what I had come to view as a relatively straightforward process of creating broth, the wife, Kathryn, boldly asked about my boobs.

"Question for you," she said with what appeared to be a sincere smile, "Do you have breast implants?"

Everyone froze. I felt the briefest glimpse of embarrassment and then a sensation that would become increasingly common in which my mind seemed detached from my body. I could almost view the scene unfolding before me as a spectator instead of a participant.

As my mind and body began to reassemble themselves, I was able to listen intently as she told us her story. Kathryn, who was the subject of a cable television episode on implant illness, shared the psychological and physical symptoms that had tortured her and had threatened to rip apart her family before she understood that her toxic breast implants were to blame.

And then it hit me—a full-body experience that I can only describe as visceral. Memories began to flood my awareness as if a dam holding back a river of "we told you so" had shattered. Some part of my brain had known all along that putting these synthetic bags of silicone inside me would not be copacetic with my fragile body. My logical mind had found a way to ignore the accumulated years of internal cautionary signals, the warning bells that had begun sounding back when I was a teenager.

As I had watched my high school friend's mother recover from her second round of implants, I had sworn that I would never mutilate myself in the name of beauty.

Implants had a shelf life of a decade if you were lucky back then (something that hasn't changed with all the advances in plastic surgery technology). I had seen vivid images of fluid and blood-filled tubes peeking out from beneath her baggy shirt while she rested in pain on the sofa for days after the procedure. These images are as clear in my mind now as they were to my fourteen-year-old self then.

But not too long after moving to our picture-perfect suburb of Jacksonville in 2010, I had found myself getting swept up in the allure of enhancing my physical appearance to keep up with the women around me. When several close friends decided to have the procedure, I joined them. Breastfeeding two kids had left me even smaller than my pre-pregnancy size 32B bosom. I found every which way to justify having a pair of "natural-looking" silicone sacks stuffed underneath my chest wall muscle. This seemingly minor surgery would give me the confidence I needed to go to the gym, wear a bathing suit, fill in those dresses I had worn when pregnancy hormones and breastfeeding had given me briefly what my genetics never had.

When I entered the fancy modern office with large floor-to-ceiling windows overlooking the lush Florida landscape below, I allowed the doctor to lead and I followed like an obedient puppy. It's tough not to feel vulnerable standing topless in front of a man in a white coat. His "expert" assurances that I would look proportionate again had left me feeling both hopeful and defective at the same time. The undertone that I would remain disproportionate without this surgery was evident. Yes, I was flat-chested, and, yes, I could look womanly with his care. He had hundreds of happy and whole patients. This is what I heard as I stood staring out the window, trying not to meet his gaze after he had become more familiar with my breasts than I was myself.

I convinced myself that my concerns at the time about the foreign silicone objects becoming an additional burden on a body that was possibly immunocompromised had been overwrought. *Women did this all the time! And what about breast cancer? Reconstruction with implants is the norm. If they can do it, I can do it. I just catch a few extra colds every now and then. Otherwise, I'm healthy,* I had told myself, despite all evidence to the contrary.

And the fears dissipated, just like that. They were replaced by hope and excitement. Maybe my inner knowing was trumped by an outer aesthetic so strong and obtrusive that the little, loving voice of integrity had no chance. A few weeks later, I had the surgery with no complications except that I was filled with a C cup instead of the more modest full B that I had requested.

"The smaller implants didn't fill you out well enough, so I went with the larger end of the spectrum we discussed," he had said as I awoke nauseated from my anesthesia-induced slumber. His comment barely registered at the time, but once I was home, I felt as though I would topple over from my new chest and its post-surgery swelling. I cannot help but wonder if a female surgeon would have found that my requested B cups fit me perfectly.

While the pain and swelling were manageable, the loss of "me" was strangely difficult. Sure, I did feel a boost of confidence in clothes. But if I disliked looking at my naked flat chest in the mirror before, I hated looking at my new chest now. Not only were the faux boobs weirdly disconcerting, but my breast skin was so delicate and translucent that I could see the rippling of the ripple-resistant implants. It was not surprising that sleeping on my stomach became uncomfortable with the enhancement.

"Why are you still wearing a bra to bed?" Matt asked one night, six months after the surgery, as I pulled a soft and tattered tee shirt over the sports bra I had been wearing all day to harness my boobs in place.

I was wearing a bra because my chest still felt like I had those painfully engorged breasts of my infant-feeding days. What I did not anticipate was the fear that they would pop with any additional pressure; the implants seemingly so close to the surface of my skin and all. I had to wonder why he stuffed mangoes in a space made for a pair of plums.

◎ ◎ ◎

Here with Laura and her clients, I was once again in a room full of strangers examining my breasts. *So much for being the authority.* I was instead back to being the sick patient. This conversation, focused on me and my failing body, quickly thwarted my enthusiasm about being a health mentor and having the opportunity to give back to others.

My three-year boob experiment came to a close shortly after the comment in the kitchen that day. Taking out the toxic bags seemed imperative at this point, so I decided to contact this woman's surgeon. My husband and I opted to drive to Georgia for the procedure, knowing that we would come home twelve thousand dollars poorer but hopefully richer in optimism. *Can't put a price on that,* we thought, rationalizing this next hefty health-seeking expense.

When I awoke from the surgery, my husband was beside me, reassuring me that all had gone well. As someone who now made a living as a surgical sales representative, Matt appeared genuinely impressed listening to the doctor recount how two surgeons meticulously removed the implants, capsular scar tissue lining, abnormal scar tissue, and infected lymph nodes that were afflicting me. The implants, which had taken all of fifteen minutes to stuff under my chest muscles three years ago, took two surgeons four hours to remove.

Back then I had remained hopeful that this latest magic pill would be the one. I had experienced bouts of relief under the care of my functional medicine doctor but most were short-lived. A week of renewed energy or a clear head on the heels of a dietary or supplement modification was always followed by a relapse into the same dis-ease. I was never unstuck for long. After almost two years of unexplainable fatigue, digestive distress, erratic and debilitating pain, brain fog, and a laundry list of bizarre symptoms, this had to be it.

But it wasn't.

The post-surgery antifungals and antibiotics had duped me. As my drug-induced honeymoon came to an end, so did my optimism. I found myself once again trapped in a body plagued by an internal war.

I remember a few months later when Matt and I traveled southwest, no kids in tow for once, down the Sunshine State, and I could do nothing but cry uncontrollably.

We drove from northeastern Florida to the Gulf Coast city of Sarasota that we would soon call home. Matt had recently accepted a promotion that required a move from the state's east coast to the west—from the region of Florida that still experiences a semblance of four seasons to the small town that attracts snowbirds and rarely sees temperatures below 50° F.

I had been crying for three hours and counting. I did not even know why I was crying. That realization did not change the fact that I was unable to make it stop. My patient and loving husband's words of comfort, the peaceful drive through lush canopy tree-lined roads of inland Florida, the upbeat music heard from the satellite radio— none of it could dig me out of that deep, dark hole.

As someone who had never experienced depression, I can now say with conviction that this condition is not all in your head. I gained no respite from thinking happy thoughts, trying to snap out of it, or looking on the bright side. I found little comfort in the company of another person. Depression is lonely. Having someone who loved me deeply by my side did not wash away the emptiness I felt within me, even if I hoped it would.

A part of me, some barely perceptible loving part of me, must have watched the scene, unable to step in and pull me up. The sadness prevailed. The tears ran wild like a broken fire hydrant on a peaceful sidewalk. I was sure all anyone could see was the damaged shell of a person I felt I was. In that moment, I wanted my husband to wrap his arms around me and reassure me that I was loved, but how could I let him in when I wasn't even sure that I loved myself?

This is the hypocrisy that my mind created when I was depressed—I wanted comfort but couldn't reach out for it.

When we arrived at the first house to meet our Realtor, I should have been giddy with anticipation. I love change. I love house hunting. I love the novelty of creating a new living space. But that day, my body felt too weak to stand, and my mind was too jumbled to engage. I somehow managed to go through the motions by avoiding eye contact and small talk. My sunglasses, worn both outdoors and in, created the barrier I felt I needed to protect everyone from seeing my brokenness. I quickly scanned the dozen or so houses on our tour, each time rushing back to the comfort of my seat in the car. My husband did the house hunting for both of us, while I struggled to feel alive.

Although I was fortunate not to add long-term depression to my growing list of symptoms, I was coming to terms with the fact that the explant surgery had not been my magic pill. However, as subtle a shift as it was, I felt that I was making progress in accepting myself, aesthetic flaws and all. Having the beauty-enhancing implants removed sent a powerful message to my body that we are in this together. With the heavy silicone-filled sacks out of me, I felt surprisingly free. Free to sleep on my stomach again—a luxury I had taken for granted until it was gone. Free to take deep breaths without feeling like I was pushing a set of sandbags off my chest. Free to move and breathe and dance through life as *me*, unencumbered.

It took a life-endangering surgery and tens of thousands of dollars to understand that happiness cannot be bought and plastered on my chest. Sure, I had felt more confident in clothing. Every style of shirt seemed to cling to my torso beautifully, and shopping for blouses had become a hobby for a while, literally. My husband would say, without an ounce of criticism in his voice, "My hobby is fly fishing. Yours is online shopping." He never guilted or shamed me about it. He also never pushed me into getting my augmentation in the first place. He had simply supported my decision. Poor guy never benefited from them either because I was too ashamed of their inauthenticity to show him. Not feeling like me was worse than embodying the real me, flat chest and all. After several months of healing from this second round of surgery (the mango-sized sacks removed and the weird rippling nice and smooth again) Matt was able to see his wife's unclothed chest once more. And I was actually kind of happy with it.

The thing about the neuroplasticity practices I was incorporating into my life as I headed into 2016 was that they naturally guided me back to my authenticity. The most effective mantras and visualizations were the ones in which I was unencumbered by any desire to please another person or wear some sort of mask to fit in. Reliving experiences of feeling my toddler's arms around my neck and cheek upon my chest, sitting with my husband on the deck of a fancy hotel overlooking a majestic cliffside ocean, or walking through the front door of my grandmother's house and into her outstretched arms—these all felt effortless. In those moments all was good.

CHAPTER 12

Wounded Healer

AS I MADE MY WAY THROUGH THE COURSEWORK FOR my master's degree in nutrition, I naturally gravitated toward the macro and micronutrients material and hands-on cooking labs. Research and statistics, nutritional history, and even the organic chemistry pre-req I was required to take all fueled my naturally curious desire to understand the origin of this "food as medicine" concept better.

But my insistence on finding the perfect diet as my primary means to heal fostered a new problem: Orthorexia, obsessive behavior centered around a healthy diet, was brewing inside me. I had a compulsive need to control not only my diet, but those of my kids, too. That summer, I wrote to my sons' camp director with concerns about the sugary snacks and drinks given to the kids each evening. I outlined my older son's diet, detailed particulars of his immune system, and even included scientific studies. I went so far as to suggest what foods the camp should provide to the kids (to which the camp director replied and politely declined). Attempting to control my sons' camp experiences was just one externally focused manifestation of this obsessive behavior.

Of course, the focus of this mania was me. The scarcity mentality I had begun to adopt after years of restrictive dieting was manifesting in a few troubling ways. While the carbohydrates added back into my routine after my failed keto attempt felt like liberation, this newfound freedom was still tainted with anxiety to the point of being pissed off when someone ate my gluten-free bread or healthy granola bar (which could be easily replaced by a two-minute drive to the grocery store).

"Oh no you don't," I would growl at my husband, snatching the last vegan, Paleo, macrobiotic bar in the house from his hand.

"How about this Clif bar? Is this one safe for me to eat?" he would ask, scanning the fine print on the nutrition label. "It looks like there's wheat in this thing, so you can't have it anyway."

"Yes. You know I can only eat these," I indicated as I held up my now taped up chocolate sunflower butter bar. "And what happens if I'm out tomorrow, and I get weak and hungry? I have to have something safe to eat." I held onto certain foods as if my life depended on them.

There was another mark in this scarcity imprint that I was just starting to recognize. My disorder and the desperation to heal had, at their core, a feeling of unworthiness that was being temporarily alleviated by experiencing the joy of indulging in my favorite foods. I overate healthy snacks like cleverly marketed nutrition-rich granola bars. These foods briefly filled a cup that would otherwise have been filled with emotions I did not want to swallow. Emotional distraction by way of overeating and territorializing my food were becoming real problems.

Visiting family in the mountains of North Carolina that year proved to be vexing as I began managing the overpacked car. The weeklong vacation entailed that we rent a towable U-Haul to hold all of my "safe" food ingredients and special toxin-free appliances (Vitamix, cast iron pan, and mini food processor all come to mind). Arriving in the small mountain town with all the pomp and circumstance certainly didn't make me look any less crazy to my family. I know my parents and siblings were trying to understand my illness out of genuine love and concern for me, but they were confused why I wasn't able to find meal ingredients at the local Food Lion and cook with their kitchen supplies. Afterall, they didn't live in a log cabin in the woods! If I was being rational, I would have realized that surviving on non-organic produce and GMO-laden dry goods was actually feasible. Fear had smothered my rational mind.

My obsession with food now officially out of control, I wondered if it was time to rethink my plan to complete a master's in nutrition. Perhaps the coursework was partly driving my compulsion to eat only the "right" foods. Besides, I found that when things got too technical, I checked out. One day in early 2016, while I sat at my computer registering for my second nutritional biochemistry and pathophysiology course (topics that, unfortunately, didn't hold my attention as much as I had hoped), I wandered onto a page with some much more appealing course options. I started seeing words like mindfulness, meditation, and psychoneuroimmunology.

Wait a second, I thought. *I don't remember these courses being available in the program. Have they added more electives?*

I scrolled to the top of the web page and realized I had inadvertently navigated to the Master of Health and Wellness Coaching section of the university's website. I could not help but feel that I was being somehow divinely guided to this path. These courses seemed to closely correlate with the neuroplasticity practice that had become so integral to my healing. I did a little research, made a few phone calls, and within a week transferred my applicable credits to this new degree track. I was on my way to attaining an education that was better suited to my future career.

❂ ❂ ❂

Shortly after switching degrees, I read about a woman named Martha Beck. She was apparently Oprah Winfrey's expert life coach at one time and a master at helping people break down the walls of their ingrained social constructs to find the hidden compass within. She also trains "wayfinders" to become coaches in all areas so that they, too, can help others navigate life more easily. Wayfinders, according to Martha, possess a set of unique characteristics, a few of which include the desire to be part of a transformational human mission, abundant empathy, an extroverted yet solitude-yearning personality, chronic physical illness, and an emotional connection to animals that differentiates them from most others. This sounded a lot like me.

I followed the breadcrumbs that were being tossed along the path before me. A free informational call about Martha Beck's eight-month coach training program happened to be scheduled later in the week, so I made it a priority to be there.

As luck (or fate?) would have it, Martha took my question on the group call. After hearing about the logistics of the program and feeling a growing sense of urgency to add this training to my growing autodidactic toolkit, I asked for her take on the subject of neuroplasticity. While she had not used this word in the overview, the excitement in her voice made it clear to me that the methods she teaches are intricately woven into the notion that the brain is elastic and able to change itself. In response to my description of several debilitating illnesses, she told us about her diagnosis many years before of fibromyalgia. In less than five minutes, she helped me shed my beliefs about my limitations by offering a novel perspective on my body's health decline.

"Have you heard of shaman sickness?" she asked. I could hear a story about to unfold, and I sat expectantly.

She then described the role of the healer in certain Indigenous cultures. In many shamanic societies, she explained, it is believed that when a member of the tribe is challenged by persistent or recurring illness, the way to heal is through healing others. Once that person steps back into alignment with their purpose as healer, their disease is no longer "needed." The suffering they experienced prepares them to align with their true purpose and better serve others.

As Martha spoke, goosebumps appeared on my arms as I felt a chill of recognition. Of all the modalities I had sampled, of all the diets I had mastered, of all the research I had done, the idea of healing myself so that I could help others felt as true to me as my love for my children. It just made sense. Reflecting on the past year or so, I could see how my body came alive and any resonance of illness quieted whenever I was able to share what I had learned about health and healing with others. Renewed energy seemed to magically appear out of nowhere when the opportunity arose to mentor a neighbor through a moldy house crisis or help a family member implement healthful dietary changes.

After the call, I began to ponder this idea of the wounded healer, and you probably have already guessed what I did next: some online research. I found that Carl Jung, a forefather of modern psychology (and Jungian analysis), spoke frequently about the wounded healer archetype, one who is able to focus on the suffering of others rather than their own. Like the chronically sick member of Indigenous societies who steps into the role of healer, I felt that in giving advice to others, I was telling myself what I continually needed to hear. And where I continued to struggle with afternoon exhaustion and brain fog, my words to others served as fresh reminders for healing myself.

I was beginning to recognize that these painful few years had been and were continuing to transform me. Without sickness I would not have gone to such great lengths to change my lifestyle habits and protect my family from food and environmental toxins. My motivation to pursue the new master's degree direction and follow the tracks to this complementary life coach training was a testament to the increasing energy I enjoyed at the thought of helping others. I felt joy and a zest for life that had been dormant for decades before the DNRS workshop had planted the seeds for this ever-growing mind-body path. I was healing. I could feel it in my core. I got the sense that all I was doing now in preparation to serve others would also help me uncover the emotional blocks to my physical recovery.

The idea of serving others dovetailed nicely with the brain rewiring training and lifestyle changes I had been putting in place. It seemed like this concept of neuroplasticity was quickly becoming a central focus of my healing path and could be the way in which I would be able to serve others on theirs. The scientist in me continued to want to understand it and find ways to explain it—first to my friends and family and eventually, God willing, to future clients as I would help them learn to embrace this courageous form of healing as well.

I began to see and explain the concept to others in this way: Imagine a well-trodden path through the woods that leads you through your day. You are immediately drawn to this path because it is familiar, cleared of shrubs and vines, and comfortable to walk. You have walked it a thousand times. This path does require you to cross a bridge over a swampy pond and traverse some prickly weeds, but you no longer have to think about it or trouble yourself with the risks of finding another way. Like the movie *Ground-hog Day,* you keep reliving the same walk over and over. It takes tremendous dedication to choose the new route, but you finally decide to do it.

One day, you face your fears and forge a new path through the woods. This is not such an easy task. It requires a machete to hack through vines, enormous strength to move boulders, and endurance to climb the steep hills. You explore this alternate path. Maybe today you stop yourself before getting angry at your husband for not getting the right organic, grass-fed meat. Instead, you take a deep breath and let it go. At least he was kind enough to make a special trip to pick up the groceries. But the next day you find yourself resigned to taking the easy route once again— the quick temper, over-identifying with symptoms (*woe is me*), living in a protective bubble to keep the toxic world out, letting illness identity run rogue in your psyche. The well-worn path is just so enticing that it is automatic, but it also does not feel as good at the end of the day because you experience the same problems and fail to see the potential for something new and better. Eventually, as you continue your laborious practice of coming back to this untraversed path you start to notice soft grass for your feet and pretty flowers adorning the sides. Your day is ultimately more pleasant along this route, but it took time and attention to create it. As you begin to travel this path more and more, the original, easier one becomes overgrown with weeds and less enticing.

The brain's neural pathways are like the various paths through the woods: Some are well-trodden and can be traveled along with ease. Many more are blocked by the cumbersome branches, steep inclines, and rocky boulders of an unclear or unexperienced expanse of forest. Some are created out of early habits that have become ingrained and others materialize over time. It may seem crazy that the brain would choose to cause physical pain, GI distress, or fatigue in response to a trigger, but remember that the brain, like a foot traveler, is continuously seeking the path of least resistance, the well-worn and well-known path. It initially created this path in an attempt to protect you from what it perceived as a threat. The trail was paved with good intentions, but over time, the path became worn and smooth and inviting even though it no longer served you well.

Put even more simply, you can think of these as mental muscles. Just as with physical muscles, practice and repetition are vital in strengthening them. The way you think, in effect, creates new mental muscles in your brain. Continue to think a certain way, "This sense of smell is my superpower," and those muscles will grow bigger and stronger. Reframe the negative thoughts, "My unbearable sense of smell is debilitating," and those muscles that were not serving you will get weak as new healthier muscles take their place.

CHAPTER 13

At Your Service

AS I DOVE INTO MARTHA BECK'S COACH TRAINING program while wrapping up the last few classes of my master's degree in early 2017, I was beginning to feel more self-aware. I knew that if I was to become a truly effective health practitioner, I needed to be authentic. In other words, I needed to be healthy myself—mentally, physically, and spiritually. Having experienced pain, I could be a wounded healer. Now I wanted to be an example for my clients and doing so demanded that I continue to work on healing myself.

I was on a group call with Martha Beck when I experienced a lightbulb moment. My most persistent symptom was debilitating fatigue, and Martha pressed me to investigate it. "Can you find your fatigue and exhaustion right now?" she urged me on the call that day. "From one to ten, with zero being no energy at all and ten being bouncing out of your skin with effervescence and the desire to move, where are you today?"

Finding my fatigue sounded like something out of the twilight zone—the idea of ascribing a number to something as amorphous and pervasive as feeling tired was such an obscure request. My fatigue was too much a part of me to separate into something I could rate.

"Seven," I managed to say, barely more audible than a whisper.

"Okay, we're going to work with that. Find a slight tiredness that you're living in right now. Can you go there?" she asked me. I was still reeling from the fact that my question had been selected among dozens to be the central focus of this quarterly live call with the queen of personal growth.

"Yes," I responded.

"Focus on the fatigue. See the fatigue as a being that lives in your body. It's not Carrie. It's a feeling that affects Carrie. Switch between you and your fatigue. This is an imagination game."

"Okay," I said. *Have we gone over this coaching technique in class yet? I'm a good student if not,* I told myself. I could pretend to get this. I mean, I kind of got it.

Martha continued with her visualization activity. "I want to talk to the fatigue as if she's a separate person, and the classic way to do this in Jungian analysis is to switch chairs. You will be the fatigue sitting in chair #1 and Carrie in chair #2. Can you get into character as your fatigue? Being your fatigue?"

"Yes." Okay, this was getting more bizarre by the minute, I thought, and now I was feeling performance anxiety to boot. How could I "get into character" with only about a hundred other coaches-to-be listening intently to this dialogue?

"Get into character and start giving me descriptions from inside. 'I am the fatigue. I am heavy. I am sluggish. I am frustrating.' But be sure you don't switch back into being Carrie. Be the fatigue itself."

"How are you doing today, fatigue?" she offered, starting off this dialogue in her bubbly, childlike voice.

"I am . . . uh, mud in her veins," I (the fatigue) answered back.

"Carrie's veins. I am mud in Carrie's veins," she interrupted.

"I am mud in *Carrie's* veins. I am sleepy. I am draining Carrie," I said. I was getting the hang of this.

"Fatigue, how are you trying to help Carrie? Don't think it through. Just blurt it."

I tried not to think too hard. "I am calming her down. I am stopping her."

"Let me ask you this," Martha nudged a bit more. "Fatigue, how do you feel about Carrie?"

"I love her." Sappy, Trite. Did this fatigue being really say that or did I . . . um, Carrie, say it for her/it?

"I love her. I'm calming her." Huh . . . okay.

"Fatigue, do you have any messages you've been trying to get through to Carrie? Would you like to say what you've been wanting to tell her, please?" Martha really wanted to keep beating a dead horse, it seemed.

I let out a long sigh. "I'm here to bring her back."

Where the heck did that come from?

"I'm here to bring *you* back," she corrected me.

Oops. "I'm here to bring *you* back," said the fatigue.

"Just say it to her, please." Her guidance was kind and loving, albeit a bit nerve-wracking. I felt there was so much at stake as I sat there in the virtual spotlight.

"I'm here to bring you back . . . I'm here to put you on the right path. I'm here to help you connect?" I said/asked. The words were coming to me without too much logical left-brain thought. Still, I was also keenly aware that all ears were on me, so it was tough to remain entirely in character.

"Uh, huh. Connect with what? With whom?" she prodded.

"Yourself. I'm here to help you feel. To be present," I continued. Trite again. But it felt strangely true.

"The culture doesn't encourage us to be present. It encourages us to ignore the internal signals," she said, returning her attention to "Carrie" now. "You're being told, Carrie, that you're supposed to live a certain life. And you've bought the whole package because you're a high achiever. Tell me where I'm wrong."

"I am. And it's hard when that fatigue hits because sometimes I'm enjoying being a high achiever." There was that familiar energetic voice that accompanied the euphoria I felt when I was high and achieving.

"Why would you not?" Martha exclaimed with shared excitement in her voice. "You get all kinds of strokes! But being a high achiever means achieving things that your ego values. Oh, it feels so good to be admired and see all this work piling up and to tell myself I am productive today. I am excited about this. Of course, it feels good. You've been taught that that's what should make you feel good. What you haven't had is a friend who will forcibly hold you down, slow you down, calm you down, and tell you there's guidance coming from somewhere else—like finding things that give you joy that you may never have even known existed."

My body is my friend? What nonsense is this?

"The only reason, Carrie, that you and I are talking like this is that I have chronic pain," Martha continued. "Without that teacher, I would probably be a tenured professor somewhere grinding out stupid journal articles that no one reads and trying to get prizes."

Her words helped me understand that her chronic pain was my fatigue. We both endured the burden of these bodily teachers so that we could find meaning in life that we would not have otherwise been able to discover.

While I had her full attention, I asked, "Well, what do you do when you feel like you're following your North Star (your flow, your intuition, your divine guidance) and you're doing something that you think really is fueling your soul, but then the pain or the fatigue hits? I can be out in nature, doing something that I know has to be good for me, and it hits."

"Ah, you said you know that it has to be good for you," she replied, picking up on cues that my logical mind was trying to make my body out to be the enemy again, not benefitting from what common sense would say is best for it. "There are times when taking a walk is self-destructive. I'm working right now with a person who's in severe adrenal burnout who is used to taking long walks in the woods. Her doctor said to her, 'If you took walks in the woods every day, you would get cancer or diabetes or a heart attack. You are at such a level of exhaustion that you should be sleeping ten hours a night plus two naps a day. No exercise until we've got your numbers better. Do not go for a walk in the woods.' And her whole body just sagged with relief because that was the inner message. As soon as she stopped trying to go for walks in the woods and gave herself permission to sleep she began healing rapidly."

I moved from the pair of chairs in my office where I had been playing the roles of "fatigue" and "Carrie," and fell onto the white slipcovered sofa with its down pillows and cozy chenille blanket. I sank into the tranquility of this moment, allowing the soft furnishings to gently embrace me. It felt magical to have been given permission to truly let go.

"The culture doesn't have the answers." I closed my eyes and allowed her words to settle into my psyche. I sensed this session was coming to a close, and I wanted to absorb every last morsel of her wisdom. "And this is true even when everything is screaming at you, 'Get something done because it's the only way to feel good!' What you need to do in those moments of fatigue is really look inside your body. Stop making the fatigue the enemy. It came from you. It said it loves you, and it's trying to guide you.

"Your body, your essential self, your animal has the compass. Your social self doesn't have the compass. If you'd been raised by criminals, you would be a high-achieving criminal, and that wouldn't make it right—just because everyone around you said 'Yes, that's achievement.'

"Your fatigue is speaking to you. It's guiding you. It's a friend. It's love. And it will rip you away from culture, like my son ripped me away from culture, and made me find myself."

The son she referred to has Down syndrome and is the subject of one of my favorite books, *Expecting Adam*.

She paused for a moment and then continued, "The body is an animal. Be kind to animals. It's a horse that knows the way home in a blizzard. You think it's going in the wrong direction, but it knows better than the mind. The mind is crazy. The body knows its way home."

My body felt more at peace in that moment than it had felt in quite a while. My head melted back on the sofa cushion. My tight shoulders and clenched gut let up a bit, along with the bars of the cage I had constructed to protect my heart. I was now completely oblivious to others on the call. Maybe that was also because they, too, were entranced. It was just me, Martha, and the wise bodily vessel that seemed to contain the sensations of this moment. Fatigue did not feel angry. It was not defective or frail. It was soft and calm. Centered and grounded. It felt like home.

"For you, the gift is coming in the form of fatigue. When you love your fatigue, fully, then I'll believe you're really getting its messages. When you love it as much as it loves you. The body self says, 'No fear, be calm, trust, surrender.' And my mind says, 'But I don't want to! I want to be sure that everything's going to be okay!' And the body says, 'Right now everything is okay. There is nothing but right now. Surrender.' Very strong medicine. Can you do it? Can you redefine achievement so that this is the way you do well?"

Deep in my soul, I knew that was what was necessary to get me out of the pit I was in. Buried below all the weariness and fog, the anxiety and physical pain, there was arrogance at the core. It believed that I should not still be sick, yet suffering is clearly part of our shared human experience. I had so easily forgotten that my timeline, my efforts, my plan to make it through this rough patch by now was not the divine plan. I had acted as though I did not know that horrible things were happening to all kinds of people in every moment and that I was the only one experiencing pain. My disease had simply been a burden that I no longer wanted to bear. I had denied that my illness could be some sort of beacon calling me home to myself.

The word surrender seemed so vague to me—a word reserved for spiritual types and their ethereal like-minded groupies. I knew it involved trust, but I had never been one for trusting much of anything or anyone other than my will. I had survived the past forty-one years by creating a safe environment around me, born from my stellar ability to control everything—my childhood accomplishments, my career success, my family life, our home, our children, my health . . . well, maybe not that one. But I continued to push my agenda on my body and its failings. I felt confident my methods would work. My strategies would protect and save me as they always had.

"How is your body right now?" she asked me.

"Soft, calm . . . flowing," I responded. No need to fake it. This was truly how I felt. The tranquility coursing through my veins was in stark contrast to the mud that had filled them just minutes before.

"And as you love it, it takes you into the river. The body loves the river. And the river is spirit, and spirit is everything. And when you're connected to everything, you can do everything. But not the way our culture says. Not even the way our religions say it. I am feeling such a sense of stillness from you, Carrie, that it puts me at peace. There is a field of peace generated around you right now, and it is exquisite."

◎ ◎ ◎

Not too long after Martha spoke to me of surrender, I found myself wondering, to whom or to what was I supposed to surrender? What did it mean to trust, exactly? I felt as though I had been naive for four years in *trusting* that I would get my life back when I finally found the right healing approach, but I had not. Look where trust had gotten me!

And surrender. I was forced to surrender every single day as I stumbled to my knees, collapsed in exhaustion after more than one or two simple tasks. Finding myself stuck inside an achy, exhausted, volatile body, I had been forced to do nothing else but surrender.

Before our long phone session that day, I had asked Martha what to make of the feeling that my soul, mind, and body were detached from one another. I often felt so ungrounded when I had brain fog.

She said, "Your mind thinks it's separate from your essential self. The mind can say 'I'm all alone here.' The soul knows it is always connected to everything—that grounding cannot be taken from you. You can only imagine that it's gone because your mind believes an untrue thing, and there's a sense that you are separate from reality.

"The mind is something you can work with to end separation. The mind says, 'I'm in pain.' And then it hangs on to that. When the thought goes away, the pain goes away."

Fatigue was my body's continuous whisper to surrender and relinquish my death grip on control. My thoughts about fatigue were always more dreadful than fatigue itself. It would take me years of hearing messages such as this before I fully embraced them. Still, it was clear that surrender was a significant component of my healing path. As I let go and accepted the fatigue, instead of resisting and fearing it, its grasp on me eventually loosened. When I allowed the current of life, my body, my illness to carry me until I settled into a peaceful pool, and then felt the pull of the tide to continue on my journey, that was when I knew I had learned to surrender. Every time.

◉ ◉ ◉

As I looked for tools to help me truly let go, I began to examine my dreams. Until recently I had not been retaining the details of the stories taking place in my subconscious. Experts say that most of us dream four to six times per night and that these visions during REM sleep can last from a few seconds to thirty minutes.

I set an intention to remember my dreams, and I kept a journal and pen beside my bed. I found that I was often awoken abruptly on the heels of a fascinating dream with the urge to go to the bathroom or a brief yet sharp pain or a loud sound that no one else heard. It was as if I were being awakened on purpose so that I could indeed record these nonsensical scenes on paper. At first, the fatigue was too overwhelming, and in my half slumber, the dreams did not seem unreal (like dreams) at all. They seemed entirely logical, so I simply rolled over and went back to sleep. In time, though, I was wise enough to realize that what felt ordinary in that moment would likely seem remarkable when I was fully awake, and I continued to train myself in this way.

I had always believed that dreams of falling meant that the person felt insecurity, anxiety, or a loss of control in some aspect of her life. This blanket interpretation of a universal dream experience is like telling someone that if they crave pickles and ice cream that they must be pregnant. My dream represents a path to a core part of myself, and by investigating the various players in my distinct stories, I could get closer to my core.

When I learned to pay attention and take a little time to unravel my dreams, I realized they could be a window into my subconscious mind—a colorful emotional inner sanctuary. The education I had been receiving, both in school and through the coach training, generally aligned with Jungian theory. Imagery presented to our minds in sleep is made of symbols that help us make sense of situations or solve problems we face in our conscious state, according to Jung. So, a dozen people with the same dream scenario (like standing naked on the street) can garner a dozen different meanings, depending on the life history and associations of each dreamer. I started to learn how to interpret many of my dreams by viewing the various players—people, objects, locations, even emotions felt—as different parts of myself disconnected from my conscious mind.

The recalling of my dreams was now becoming a gateway to my emotions. Much of the "work" of processing these often locked up, stuffed down, pushed away emotions could be accomplished without my active engagement. However, I found that when I was able to hold onto the string of that last dream-filled balloon, and ever so gently pull it back to my semi-conscious state, I was able to recall them. Reflecting on these slumber-enhanced mind adventures allowed me access to an otherwise locked fantastical inner world.

Experts have found that the more theta brain wave activity in the prefrontal cortex after waking, the more likely your dreams can be remembered. Theta is that deeply relaxed state achieved just before we nod off, during REM sleep, and just before we wake up. To enhance this ability, I discovered that it's best *not* to instantly turn on my cell phone or start up a conversation with my husband. Simply by staying in this slower paced, more relaxed brain state as long as possible, I was more likely to pull those whimsical stories back before they floated away.

Since I'd found that working with a maladapted limbic system was a key component to healing from mystery illnesses, it seemed like a good idea to have a concept of how this part of the brain is affected during sleep. This is what I picked up from Martha Beck's teachings on the subject and from a little bit of online intermediate digging into the mechanics of dreams:

During REM sleep, when our neocortex (involved in higher functions like conscious thought and language) begins firing a neuronal dialogue with our hippocampus (in charge of learning, emotions, and forming new memories), we can process emotions. When the prefrontal cortex (the part of our brain that thinks critically) temporarily goes to sleep itself, other parts of our brain, namely the amygdala, can step in with unfettered access. The almond-shaped amygdala lights up and is able to process emotions more freely.

Learning to look at otherwise repressed emotions is an integral part of healing from dis-ease. When sleep is chronically disrupted, some of this innate regenerative ability is impaired. This doesn't mean all is lost. There are many proactive ways to unlock carefully guarded repressed emotions—even if you've tossed out the key, as I had throughout much of my childhood—and I would explore these soon.

◎ ◎ ◎

At this point, though, I was sleep-deep into the world of dreams. While I had several journals filled with nonsensical dream fragments, this particular one had an ample amount of emotional charge, so I chose to play with it.

I let the bus go into a parking lot. It goes through the strip mall cafe window. I am filled with guilt and feel that I need to confess. My mother sings a song to me with my father nearby, in front of a picture of my grandparents. They know. My son reenacts the scene but it becomes a water setting—the bus fills with water and he escapes . . .

except when he reenacts it again, this time horsing around and never floating up. He laughs and then says he is weak. He starts to drown.

I emerged from this twisting and turning dream feeling some intense emotions. I woke up horrified, heart racing, beads of sweat dripping from my forehead and onto the pillowcase. The overwhelming guilt I felt upon allowing the bus to drive through the cafe window was the first memory I sustained of that unusually accessible dream.

In going with the Jungian theory route to dream analysis, I opted to explore the following symbols: the bus, the photo of my grandparents, my son, the water, and my son's laughter. Like the message Martha Beck guided me to hear from my fatigue, I listened to what each of these symbols was trying to convey.

THE DREAM'S CHARACTERS AND THEIR MESSAGES

The bus was yellow, rickety, out of control:

> *I (the bus) am not yours (Carrie) to control. I want you to understand this so that you release yourself from blame when things don't go according to your plan.*

The photo of my grandparents was worn, loved, watchful:

> *We (my grandparents) are here to make you aware of our unending presence.*

My son was carefree, childlike, happy:

> *I (my son) am your reminder to let loose and*
> *enjoy life.*

The water was heavy, overbearing, ominous:

> *I (the water) am here to show you your fear.*

My son's laughter was innocent, unsuspecting, sweet:

> *This (my son's laughter) is how surrender feels.*

THE DREAM'S MESSAGE

I let go of control as it drives into catastrophe (as fear of loss of control often does when given space in the mind to embellish). My grandparents know because they are always with me. I can feel their presence if I allow myself to do so. When I'm carefree, the scene becomes a simple game. I can escape the impending disaster or I can succumb to the fear. I am weak. Too weak to continue to hold on like this. I can make the choice to simply surrender and let go of all the fears. They're only in my mind. Surrender is innocent and sweet.

◎ ◎ ◎

It was one thing to be told that surrender and trust were paramount to my healing, but receiving this wisdom from my inner knowing—from the messages gifted to me in such a profoundly captivating way by this dream—felt more motivating.

Emotions often feel amplified in dreams. I found that feeling the fear of surrender more deeply, at my core, was something my mind and body could do while I slept. My brain could construct a make-believe scene that stripped the scary emotion from its real lived circumstances, essentially demystifying it. Visiting those difficult emotions by investigating my recent dreams cracked open a door to the scary unknown that my protective conscious self would have preferred I kept closed.

CHAPTER 14

Letting Go Enough to Let Go

IN FEBRUARY 2018, A WOMAN FROM THE DNRS workshop I attended two years earlier reached out to me via email, asking if I'd be interested in joining her on a trip to see Dr. Joe Dispenza in Mexico in June. Dr. Joe is a neuroscientist, chiropractor, and increasingly popular lecturer whose books have had a tremendous impact on my understanding of how profoundly our ingrained mental and emotional habits create our physical reality. Without too much deliberation, I made space for a weeklong workshop a few months later to fully immerse myself in his consciousness-exploring guidance.

I was continuing to see results from my DNRS practice. My head felt clearer, I had a renewed sense of joy and appreciation for life, I felt less pain and had more energy. The simple fact that I was able to consider venturing to Mexico and feel giddy with anticipation was a testament to my ability to enjoy life again. Maybe his teachings could take me the rest of the way. Maybe he could help me shed the remaining fears I wore like a hazmat suit to protect me from the ever-present environmental toxins. I was fully committed to this neuroplasticity path and ready to try out his approach in person.

I was drawn to Dr. Joe's Western science meets Eastern philosophy teachings. One of his best-known lessons shows up on his Instagram page in the form of this quote: "Your nervous system is the greatest pharmacist in the world." This spoke to me on a fundamental level given my recent lived experience. If anyone could attest to the power of the mind to heal the body, it was him. After having been hit by a Bronco going 55 mph while biking in his early 20s, he was told that extensive surgery was the only option that would save him from being paralyzed. This is when his foray into the mind-body healing work began, and with intense effort he was able to avoid both surgery and paralysis.

That June, as our shuttle approached the gates of the Grand Velas Riviera Maya in the Yucatán Peninsula, we were transported to a tropical paradise. But my rush of anticipation was slightly derailed by a nagging sense of dread about my complicated digestive tract and parasites setting up camp in my stomach. All-inclusive resorts are supposed to be safe, I reasoned, but I had been warned about the dangers of brushing my teeth with sink water or eating anything uncooked and had come fully prepared with every gut healing remedy I knew of. I had taken so many nutritional measures to overcome years of physical dis-ease, I couldn't ruin all my hard work now.

One thing I love about Dr. Joe's work, which was evident when I walked into the room filled with upwards of 800 attendees, was that his science-heavy teachings attract a wide variety of people. I wasn't immersed in a conference hall of hippies any more than I was stuck with only cerebral clinicians. I felt like I could fit in here.

The woman in cropped jeans and flip flops sitting beside me at lunch was a nutritionist from Indiana. She told me that she had been listening to Dr. Joe's meditations for almost a year and the adrenal fatigue and heavy metal toxicity she had been battling were finally under control. The jovial man who leaned over the line of chairs to introduce himself was a physician from Florida whose sister had made significant strides in overcoming her multiple sclerosis (MS) through this neuroplasticity route. I couldn't help but feel like most of the people present were more proficient in this work than I was. I could already tell I had lots of catching up to do.

Our days were a mix of listening to Dr. Joe speak animatedly about the science of elevating our consciousness to rewire our brains, periodic dance party breaks, and various guided meditations. His lectures were easy for me and my scientific mind to absorb. As for the meditations and dance parties, most of the time I felt like I was trying really hard to let go so I could . . . let go. The process felt like an intense tug-of-war. It was like my inner leopardess was not completely comfortable there and could protect me from eternal embarrassment by mocking those who let out moans of ecstasy or whose bodies writhed and jerked as if possessed by aliens.

Oh no. You're not coming unglued like that! Their behavior is entirely undignified. Keep your shit together. You're not about to lose your marbles on my watch. My inner leopardess's well-meaning growl was effective at keeping me both dignified and unable to surrender enough to really benefit from spontaneous healing or some "mystical experience."

But eventually I got tired of pulling on the leash. When I let go and fell back onto the proverbial grass in defeat and looked up at the bright blue sky above, I realized that was where the beauty had been all along—in the surrender, not in the victory. I focused on the happy memories that were powerful enough to send chills up my spine and a virtual explosion of love from my heart. These moments were often fleeting because my logical mind inevitably needed control, but I took what I could get. I let go of the rope and surrendered only when my mind decided it had had enough of holding on so tightly.

In addition to continuing my knowledge of neuroplasticity and inching my way toward this notion of surrendering, I made heartfelt connections with women and men from all over the world. At dinner one evening as I sat across the table from a British-Japanese linguist who had a penchant for lucid dreaming and an Indonesian shaman who had used his mind to heal his back, injured by a fall from a four story building, we were served a gorgeous raw salad. Up to that point, I had managed to avoid anything uncooked to protect my intestinal integrity. I made a joke about the probability of being exposed to parasites, and the linguist responded by suggesting that one's body is only inhabitable to opportunistic pathogens if the internal environment is conducive to them. Based on everything we had been learning that week, I assumed that he meant "emotionally" inhabitable. *Hmmm, hopefully that's not me.* In the meantime, I was not going to be a party pooper, so I dug in.

I sailed through that evening and the remainder of the workshop, gathering up all the magic I could. I returned home a week later feeling more present and at ease. But soon I realized I had been given another parting gift— fever, chills, and nausea. Since we had been warned that the intense focus on raising our body's energy had been known to lead to flu-like symptoms, I let weeks and then months go by while I waited patiently for my body to recalibrate. The fever and chills were transient, but the nausea didn't let up.

I felt drawn to eat bland, simple foods three meals a day for the first several weeks. Kitchari, an easily digestible dish of rice and split mung beans cooked in broth with Indian spices, offered me some relief. Anything more complex and the nausea would resurface. By mid-summer, I found myself ten pounds lighter and still slowly recovering from what traditional wisdom (aka common sense) would explain had been a hefty dose of parasites.

Six weeks later, as the digestive and physical weakness continued, I decided to consult a chiropractor. I was on vacation with the family in Colorado and my weakened state seemed to bring on a case of altitude sickness that I had never experienced on previous visits to the mountains. Now fully immersed in the world of functional and integrative medicine, I wasn't interested in seeking out mainstream care and their usual medicinal solutions. I had only been to a chiropractor a few times for various aches and pains, but I had become more appreciative of their whole-body approach to illness in recent years. The doctor I found, less than a mile from our charming third story A-frame apartment in the heart of Boulder, came with rave online reviews—great listener, excellent adjustments, tremendous dietary resource. It was worth a shot.

He treated me with digestive enzymes to restore my intestines to a state less hospitable to pathogens, systemic enzymes to promote healing throughout my body between meals, anti-parasitic herbs to target the worms, and several days of spinal adjustments to relieve the altitude-related headaches. With his help, extra rest, and double my usual intake of water, I finally made a full recovery.

I couldn't help but see the irony in the conversation I'd had with my new British-Japanese friend at that dinner in Mexico. Why had I been the only one from the workshop to spend the rest of the summer eating a bland diet of rice and soup, battling an army of parasites parading through my belly? We were all exposed to the same food. Could he have been on to something? Was my body emotionally appealing to these freeloading pathogens, or was it a biological upgrade, of sorts?

I was beginning to discover that clinically diagnosed digestive distress could be viewed through another lens—one with an emotional and even spiritual meaning. At the end of the summer, I reached out in desperation to the clairvoyant I had seen years earlier. Yes, I had become so "woo woo" by this point that the left-brain, logical Carrie began putting her faith in the messages received from a spirit medium.

During our conversation I remained open to receiving whatever guidance wanted to be shared. After several minutes of what would have been interpreted by my previous cynical self as simply New Age platitudes about personal growth, leaning into support, and trusting the cyclical nature of the healing process, she (that is to say, my "guides") told me that this particular sickness was trying to teach me to surrender. I felt I was getting there.

My clairvoyant intuitive then "saw" an image of a vacuum cleaner. The vacuum cleaner supposedly represented me as a child, sucking up the energy of others around me. She called these external energies "parasites." (Of course she did!) Apparently, I was now learning to break free from cleaning up other people's emotional and energetic messes.

"This is NOT a repeat of the past," she said. "Before, it was personal present-day healing. Now, a deeper level of healing is coming from a different place inside of you. It stems from when you were less than five years old, and the chaos around you was absorbed." Trust the process and treat myself with great gentleness were her parting words, a message that made me feel lighter—like a load of cargo had been carried off my shoulders and out to sea.

And it had. When we returned home to Florida, the altitude sickness exacerbated by my months-long gastrointestinal challenges disappeared upon hitting sea level again. Relief from the constant nausea wasn't far behind.

This latest health debacle demonstrated that if I allow myself to think outside the Western box of scientifically provable diagnoses, I could often uncover truths about my body that are far more telling.

CHAPTER 15

Bridge to My Emotions

WITH ALL THE TIME I HAD BEEN DEVOTING TO research and analysis over the past few years, I felt I was beginning to lose touch with my artistic self. As a child, I had been in love with theater and musical instruments, and as a teen and young adult I was drawn to the visual art world as well. Heading to college, I assumed I would be a theater major. But practicality won out, and a degree in economics made more sense for future job prospects. As I had entered my twenties and progressed into the banking and pharmaceutical sales careers that spanned that decade, I was able to keep the flame of those hobbies burning on the side. A wheel-throwing class at the community art studio after a long day at the bank, voice lessons once a week with an instructor at the nearby college, designing a magazine-worthy nursery while a pregnant pharmaceutical rep, these creative endeavors here and there seemed to be enough to nurture my right brain.

When my children came along, I shifted into the

stay-at-home mom career that allowed me to fully embrace my creative side by designing stationery and taking on freelance design projects. I was able to weave my passions together in such a way that kept my soul alive for most of my life—until my health took a nosedive. With little time left because of my seemingly insatiable desire for sleep, I could barely do more at that point than spend time with my family and research how to heal.

Now that I was making my way back to the surface of that deep pit of dis-ease, I was finding ways to reinvigorate the artistic side of me that ended up leading to additional unexpected benefits. One way to do this, I learned through my reading, was to tap into my inner child. At first it sounded like New Age babble to me, and my ego was quite resistant to engaging in too much of anything that didn't stem from my thinking mind. My social programming was still running on repeat in the back of my head, and it was difficult for me to overcome the ingrained dogma that adults were expected to act like adults! Creative processes like those we were naturally drawn to as children—making art, dancing, fiction reading, journaling, listening to or playing musical instruments—serve our minds and bodies in multiple ways. These activities enhance the connectivity of the brain, which creates new neural pathways and helps to elicit emotion.

As I was beginning to implement these self-awareness measures into my daily life, a friend asked me to go to a hoop dancing class. I don't think I had picked up a hula hoop since 1984! During the first class I looked like Elaine from *Seinfeld* (the one where she dances like some crazed lunatic). For once, though, I didn't turn beet red. I did not feel the urge to hightail it out the door. Instead, I laughed at myself, or with myself. I enjoyed feeling parts of my body that I had forgotten existed and the playful, exuberant emotions that came along for the ride. Form new neural pathways and strengthen the connectivity between neurons? Check. Express a few long-lost childhood emotions? Check. Check. Not so hard, right?

Listening to music, too, proved very powerful for me, especially old songs that brought back memories of events long ago: carefree childhood occasions, my first love, the births of my children, exhilaration of big accomplishments achieved.

In an effort to learn more about my father, I began to email him regularly with questions. I wanted to paint a picture of his life for a keepsake book I hoped to create. In response to one inquiry about the power of songs he sent an unexpectedly rich narrative: "*A Beautiful Morning* by The Rascals," he wrote, "brings back memories of a life filled with naive optimism—unfettered by distractions, challenges and expectations that pile on once entering college and the onset of adulthood. Memories of personal friendships, playing outdoor sports, going to the lake or the beach. In light of current day madness— ever present electronics, social media, and 24/7 news blaring and stoking the fires of a hyper-polarized state-of-the-world/country discourse, hearing that song brings on a poignant reminder of things long past. Simple lyrics, simple life. In short, the good old days." Learning what this familiar tune meant to him left me feeling a sense of daughterly love and closeness that I wanted to cultivate moving forward.

I began to scroll YouTube for other familiar music, which helped bring back happy memories. Listening to the Dave Matthews Band never failed to reawaken the wild abandon I felt during college; Eric Clapton's *Tears in Heaven* took me to my bittersweet first love and first heartbreak; and Cat Stevens' *Father and Son* placed me in a room with my church youth group during a rare moment of sadness displayed with tears I rarely let flow in public. I missed our little church community, the second home I visited twice a week for much of my child-hood, I reminisced. Surprisingly, images and emotions seemed to appear in my head like little memory bubbles. If I caught them before they popped, I could often attri-bute the wave of long-lost emotion to an actual event. If I missed the images, though, I simply allowed myself the space to ride the wave of (sometimes nostalgic, some-times uncomfortable) suppressed emotions until I was left with a sense of openness and release.

I also learned to use my superpower—my hyperactive sense of smell—to recall happy times. I had learned at one of the workshops that the sense of smell connects to the part of the brain that also controls memories and emotions, the amygdala. Using this to my advantage, when I noticed the scent of something that brought back good memories, I allowed them to flow. I didn't ignore them or simply let them slip by my conscious mind unnoticed. On one occa-sion, while on vacation in Montana, this awareness came when my husband cooked his delicious pot roast. The familiar aroma of a roast in the oven brought up instant memories of my mother, brother, and me snuggled up together on our brick red chenille couch watching an episode of *Different Strokes*. Pot roast was one of my mother's go-to meals, and even though she considers herself a poor chef, this was one dish she knew how to prepare elegantly. I can still taste the nutty sweetness of the slow cooked gravy with garlic, onion, and thyme coating the soft carrots and sense the comfort of our little family trio.

Where did my thoughts go if I observed them? What stories played from the camcorder in my mind? Whatever scenes unfolded in my mind's eye, I chose to watch and immerse myself in them. I would simply feel them. I would feel the joy and love and comfort and whatever cocktail of emotions the memories elicited.

Looking through old photos and videos was another way to take me back to those comforting moments and the warm emotions that came with them. I made a point to set aside time to just look through photo albums, family videos, and old pictures stored on disks and the family computer. I would sit with the memories. I would indulge in the feelings that coincided with those experiences.

I had learned that the more I sat with the pleasant memories, the more effectively I could "rewire" my brain. I believe the practice of focusing on pleasant memories and the emotions attached to them allowed me to truly feel again.

The scientist in me was still drawn to research. Heck, my inner scientist figured out that Western medicine doesn't have all the answers, evidenced by the fact that

I had just worked out a way to feed myself good vibes through memories. Fascinated by the intricately woven threads binding emotions to the physical body, I wanted to get my hands on more proof that this relationship did indeed exist. My latest research brought me to the work of a medical doctor who dedicated his career to understanding the root of back pain and autoimmune conditions. Dr. John Sarno's book, *The Mindbody Prescription*, proved enlightening.

A controversial figure in mainstream Western medicine circles, Dr. Sarno concluded that the majority of pain that is not tied to an acute injury or a genetic condition is linked to repressed emotions, often anger. The most important part of his protocol was that patients realize and fully accept that their pain is the body's way of distracting them from the scarier pain of their stifled emotions. As crazy as it may sound, his view was that the body uses physical pain and illness to protect you from the harsher reality of negative emotions. Could my fatigue be some sort of clever distraction by my body to help me avoid feeling the discomfort of emotions I didn't want to feel? Was my brain fog a protective mechanism to curtail access to deep sadness, shame, or fear? I didn't know if these were emotions my physical body was helping me avoid, but if I were to make a bet, I would say it was a lot easier to let my leopardess out of her cage than to let flow those very vulnerable emotions. The simple realization that my symptoms may not be part of a larger illness, and possibly only manifestations of a relatively harmless condition, compelled me follow this newfound path.

According to Dr. Sarno, the brain's strategy is to keep your attention firmly fixed on your body and unaware of the threatening feelings in your unconscious. In fact, it is not uncommon for the injury or abnormality to appear in the wrong place or at an unexpected time, like when you're resting comfortably in bed.

When my hip had been locked up and in pain toward the start of my mystery illness journey, an MRI found a tear in my hip flexor. Fortunately, I was working with a physical therapist at the time who told me that there is always something to be found on an MRI if you look hard enough. He hadn't given it a second thought. I recalled how, only a few months after the MRI findings, the pain completely shifted from that hip to the other one.

Learning to distance myself from my clinical diagnoses (which could be spot on or—more often than many of us realize—somewhat misleading) and instead lean into an acceptance that the pain could be a messenger of sorts could lead to relief of both symptoms and the condition itself. Freedom from the pain could come when I was willing to face the emotions that had been masked or diverted by this pain.

Martha Beck had helped me see how my symptoms could be messengers: The fatigue that had been taking me down for years was my body's loving plea for rest. It wanted me to let go of the self-imposed demands my mind placed on me to produce and succeed (at everything).

Now I was being asked to take this symptom awareness a step further and investigate the emotions I was potentially resisting whenever I refused to sit still and listen. So how was I supposed to access these emotions that were instrumental in shaping the way my body behaved? These unpleasant, often deeply repressed feelings were difficult to just conjure up as I tried desperately to relieve the neck pain that kept me from turning to see my kids in the back seat, or as I struggled to understand why a headache could keep me from enjoying that new guided mediation. What emotions could I have been repressing when, years ago, I was mustering the energy to make it up a flight of stairs while anchored by the ache in my legs?

This is where the acceptance of, instead of resistance to, the pain came into play. At first, listening to my body's uncomfortable signals led me to insights. The kink in the neck had come on the heels of an argument with one of the boys. The headache that popped up while listening to the angelic music and body-relaxing prompts dissipated when I learned how to surrender to the experience and let go of the mental tug-of-war: *Am I mastering this practice of being present?*

Over time, this soft and kind focus on the pain would occasionally lead to an outpouring of emotion. Sometimes I wouldn't be able to pinpoint what it meant, and that was okay. I had allowed it to flow. To transcend my suppressed emotions, I had to learn to feel *and move through them.* Allowing the expression of emotions without fixating on the stories that went along with them was key.

This may seem counter to the neuroplasticity work I was doing with my positive visualizations, but in those cases, stories were used to my advantage. They were the launch pads to the felt sense of reliving those moments. Here, I was better served when I let the stories go.

Without the story, sadness doesn't have to have a negative connotation. Sadness can feel like the relief of coming home to the self. Crying has an inherent softness to it, a gentle (and sometimes not-so-gentle) billowing of energy that brings me to the serenity of the present moment. Learning to be with my difficult feelings without feeding a pessimistic cycle of mind chatter was an art that took time and practice. It would take years, if not a lifetime, of what I began to call "thought-dissolving" work to master.

CHAPTER 16
On a Trip

FEELING EMBOLDENED BY MY PROGRESS, IN JUNE 2019 I decided to try an experiment that was way outside my comfort zone. I had recently read a book by food journalist, Michael Pollan, entitled *How to Change Your Mind: What the New Science of Psychedelics Teaches Us About Consciousness, Dying, Addiction, Depression, and Transcendence.* His research and first-hand accounts of the healing potential of psychedelics on the mind and body had become a bridge into further research. What I discovered was that ayahuasca is a psychedelic made from a combination of plants native to the Amazon Basin that contains the natural hallucinogen known as dimethyltryptamine (DMT). Used in controlled settings, and not recreationally, psychedelics like ayahuasca and psilocybin were finding their place among other holistic therapies for everything from post-traumatic stress disorder to addiction to migraines. The medicines help us view our problems or traumas through a different lens by intercepting the repetitive stories we have come to believe as truth. They temporarily disable the part of the brain that keeps us trapped in our emotionally charged beliefs that create our identities, aka our egos.

I was determined to learn how to surrender. I wanted to get past the fear of letting go. A friend assured me that she had just the elixir and invited me to a quaint coastal Oregon town with the promise of an experience I wouldn't regret—the healing power of ayahuasca. For courage, I enlisted a childhood friend to go along and try it with me. Once I committed to the trip, unrelenting daily nausea began alerting me to my subconscious fears about the impending event. Unable to reconcile those fears precisely, I had been trying my best to simply acknowledge their existence and remain curious. My nervous stomach was still nagging me as I made the cross-country flight. This new experiment, which I considered part of my quest for healing, was facilitated by a woman (who will remain nameless as this practice is not sanctioned in the United States) who I knew and trusted.

We convened in a charming little airbnb house just a few blocks away from the magnificent waves and rocky shoreline of the Pacific coast. As I sat on the screened porch, I sipped my water and allowed several deep breaths to loosen my tightly wound ball of nerves. It had been about thirty minutes since I had swallowed the plant medicine, which wasn't a ceremonial brew as is custom in South America but instead a Westernized version of ayahuasca infused in a few bites of chocolate (and a much more subtle dose). Indigenous people believe ayahuasca to be the green goddess of Amazonia, or Mother Ayahuasca. She acts as your guide and can answer questions during these journeys. All you need to do is ask.

My friend had enlisted a trained guide to lead us through this experience. My hope was to uncover some of the hidden emotions that may have been holding me back from fully healing. Other than low energy, my physical symptoms of dis-ease were no longer present. But I felt a nagging sense that something was still missing. I believed there was a lightness, an I-don't-give-a-shit-ness that could inhabit a more significant part of my life if I kept progressing on this healing quest.

As I sat there alone on the porch waiting for the mystical experience to begin, I could feel that my mind was resisting the unknown. I had trouble thinking about anything other than what was about to happen. Then suddenly the fear manifested as a queasy pit in my gut and, like at that beach party years before, a thickening tongue. It had been decades since I last experienced this tongue swelling sensation after my bong adventure in college. *What? Again?* These sensations seemed to command my full attention. *How do I navigate this discomfort?* I asked with an uncertainty that there was anyone there to really answer.

And the response came immediately in the form of a profound sense of inner knowing. I was told to allow the knot in my stomach to work itself out and simply focus my attention on the images behind my eyelids. I was left unfettered to immerse myself in the experience: a vintage '80s psychedelic picture show that started with little red pulsing lights and culminated in a *Star Wars*-style outer space ride complete with G.I. Joe figures in the cockpit and all manner of celestial objects viewed from my closed eyes. I was suddenly released from the incessant tracking of my thoughts. My mind was free to see the messages of my psyche without being hindered by the rigidity of my rational brain overanalyzing the sensations of my physical body. And it was that easy. I let the fear of nausea go. When the fear was free to go, so was the discomfort itself.

I walked back inside to join the others and get comfortable with a pillow and an eye mask. The show took a turn into the beautiful world of florals and fractals. What began as a single colored flower morphed into intricate pastel candy-like landscapes. Eventually, I saw the fractal patterns of the kaleidoscopes Dr. Joe and his students often referred to during his workshops. Those images that had always felt so unattainable to me in my locked up and self-conscious state were now presenting themselves in a peaceful explosion of color. The more I had struggled at his events, the more I had seen only blackness behind my closed eyelids.

The themes of the images seemed to ebb and flow for hours before I found myself laughing out loud because I couldn't find my tongue! My logical mind was trying to find its place in this journey and wanted to check in with my lemon-like body part. But it couldn't find it. My mind searched my mouth for a tongue that was now so small it could be a raisin. And I was in awe of this irony.

Although I was finally letting go enough to sense something mystical and beyond what my conscious mind had thus far allowed, I still felt a dichotomy between this place of surrender and my need to control. Amid the experience, I was both grateful and also heard myself say, *Been there, done that. I can cross this off my bucket list now.* I wanted control of my physical body and my reliable logical mind back as I found myself drifting to sleep for the night.

Ayahuasca is all about intention, according to our guide. It is more a magnifier than a creator, as it amplifies our focus upon entering the journey. My intention that time was to open myself up to a new experience. My goal was to learn how to surrender. I found that the effects lasted long after the ceremony itself, and I continued to notice the ripples of the medicine's subconscious work in the following weeks and months. At night, my sleep was rich and restorative, and although I didn't always recall the details, my dreams left me with a sense that I had felt emotions very intensely. During the day, I felt a lightness and ability to be okay with whatever crossed my path. I hadn't felt that ease in years. My hypervigilant limbic brain, which had kept me stuck in familiar patterns and suffocating safe environments for so long, was mellowing out. It was difficult to put into words, but I felt free to live again.

Months later, once the magic of the plant medicine journey had worn off some, my reasoning, sensible mind felt the urge to do a little digging into that lemon tongue sensation. Maybe there was some logical explanation for it. Perhaps the internal messages I had gotten that night about simply releasing my fearful focus on the uncomfortable sensations and enjoying the moment were just psychedelic-induced delusion. I came across some research that linked the sensation of tongue swelling to anxiety.

Real swelling of the tongue can mean several different serious conditions, but mine was never actually swollen. The hyper sensitization that came along with my fear of surrender was heightened during both of my plant-based experiments. My anxiety about losing control was misplaced onto thoughts and feelings centered on my tongue. The mind is potent, and when my thoughts are laser-focused on the sensations of my body, my body starts to feel different. As I focus on the discomfort of a body part, the body part will respond to my command.

I do not know why my tongue had become the center of attention in college, but I was not surprised that an experience twenty-two years later triggered something similar in my subconscious that made its way to the surface of my conscious mind that night. I was able to face my fear—fear of a tongue that would get so big as to overtake my body—and see it for what it really was. Just a little body part that could do and be anything my mind told it to be. The lemon was my reminder that letting go was the only way through.

I sensed that there was more work to be done on this letting go of control thing, so I found myself back into the mind-bending work as the year progressed. With the help of a local plant medicine facilitator, these forays into my subconscious felt more like intense mental labor than any sort of leisurely play. Other plants like kanna and sassafras helped me learn to rest in the presence of my true self—a spaciousness emptied of expectation, uncertainty, and overflowing anxieties—with a depth that I hadn't been able to feel despite my years of meditations, visualizations, and neuroplasticity workshops. Each encounter chipped away at the stiff barrier protecting my inner fluidity. With the medicine's gentle support, I was able to drop the constant barrage of self-deprecating thoughts and cage-like body armor and just be free to feel the perfection of who I am. It is a feeling that is so difficult for me to describe, especially because I honestly cannot remember a time when I experienced anything that comes close. It seemed like a return to a known felt sense, but not one that I could ever truly remember experiencing in my life-time. Describing it is like trying to articulate the taste of chocolate to someone who is unaware of it. Until they experience the multi-sensory indulgent treat for them-selves, making correlations to other flavors and textures is not enough. I tried my best by telling others that in the moment it felt like four decades of cement bricks had been lifted off my chest, leaving me with a euphoria so intense that I couldn't imagine ever wading through the muck of life as I once had.

In addition to these occasional plant-imbibing cer-emonies, I revisited a modality that I had tried several years before called Tension and Trauma Release Exercise (TRE®). Created by Dr. David Berceli, TRE® is a series of exercises that assist the body in releasing your mus-cles from patterns of tension, trauma, and stress. This seemingly unusual process that often involves awkward hip thrusting and bizarre arm twitches, as well as the leg tremor on which it is based, taps into one of our most nat-ural bodily activities, I learned. We are inherently made to shake off our stresses, both physical tension and often repressed emotional cargo. We need not carry all this extra weight around with us. Not only do most of us have decades worth of energetic luggage, but we pack these bags ever heavier day after day.

This innate mechanism is commonly seen in dogs who shiver in waves on the heels of an exciting encounter, or the full body vibration women sometimes experience after the intensity of giving birth. TRE® helps initiate this built-in neurological, biological, and physiological recovery system. Deep muscle contractions designed to protect the body from harm during intense or traumatic experiences are meant to literally be shaken out once they have ended. The muscles and emotions must be released to balance the nervous system. The sympathetic fight-or-flight response is naturally followed by the limbic system's ability to achieve a relaxed state of parasympathetic rest-and-restore by tremoring. Genius!

I learned more about the connection between prolonged stress and the prevalence of modern-day ailments when I started reading neuroendocrinology researcher Dr. Robert Sapolsky's book, *Why Zebras Don't Get Ulcers*. According to this book, the reason wild animals know how to dissipate stress is that they simply shake it off and move on. Humans have been socially conditioned to stifle this natural reflex, to our detriment. Over time, the smothering of this healing flame can lead to chronic pain and physical and emotional dis-ease.

When I first discovered this modality and was given the proper instructions for fatiguing my leg muscles just enough to initiate the subtle inner tremble, I was awestruck. Before my mind pushed itself into the picture, my legs seemed to get carried away by the primitive movements of the inner psoas muscles. It felt at once novel and primal—like my body had been here before and had been craving this energetic outlet for a long time. Once my mind decided that it was weird and embarrassing, a symphony of snarky remarks ensued. *You're just making this happen. This isn't real. Stop flailing around like a fish out of water and control yourself already!*

But I stayed the course and continued to practice the shaking exercise in the following weeks. After several ten- to twenty-minute sessions, my body felt like butter and the continued pulse of gentle energy coursing through my veins was indescribably peaceful. Not long after I had begun practicing this new body-centered modality, I invested in the official training and, with fresh enthusiasm, proceeded to share it with family and friends.

My daily tremor practice expanded from a barely perceptible inner thigh quiver to full body waves of release as I became more and more comfortable in my skin. My hands would flutter; hips would bounce; sometimes my shoulders and head would even twitch—all outside of my control. It was as if my body had a mind of its own. My thinking brain just needed to shut up long enough for my body to be able to express itself freely. I allowed the physical jolts and oscillations to fully express themselves, mysterious hand motions, spontaneous dancing, and all.

I am sure these physical forms of energetic release paved the way for an unexpected middle-of-the-night vomiting episode near the end of 2019. This time, as the nausea attempted to wake me from my peaceful slumber, and my habitual response spared no effort in pushing it away, I found myself easing into a state of acceptance. With this newfound ability to face my fear of losing control, I realized the glorious feeling that ensues when I learn to surrender. The freedom that unfolds when I am simply able to say that I am willing. I am willing to let go. I am willing to face this fear. I am willing to have this experience. There is so much ease and grace in the midst of the mess. Decades of resistance had been given room to move. In less than an hour, my 39-year hiatus from puking came to an end, and I felt nothing short of victorious.

The TRE® work led to a great sense of physical release, and I found myself drawn to new forms of physical movement to give my body room to express itself. My interest in finding a dance class started with the idea that I needed a form of cardio exercise that would be more fun than walking around my sauna-like 95°+ neighborhood streets during our extended May to October south Florida summers. But as I looked online for dance fitness classes in my area and saw videos of the perfectly in sync class members, I was intimidated. I was not prepared to show up at the studio door one day and fumble my way through the hip-hop movements and cues. I needed lessons first. I needed to warm up those feet!

Salsa seemed like a good place to start. After several private lessons, my Latin ballroom instructor, Charles, began encouraging me to "feel the freedom and expansion of being grounded in my own moving energy." (Yes, apparently one can be grounded and moving at the same time!) We had been working together for months, and though I could pick up the steps and make the turns, my motions felt stiff. I was relying on the energy of this pro, ten years my junior, to pull me along. I knew this rigidity—the unwillingness to sexily sway my hips or show any semblance of exotic expression as Latin dancers so often do—was rooted in my struggle to fully let go. Much of that struggle was tied to the fear that surrendering meant looking graceful and feminine, something my inner leopardess didn't care for at all.

Charles tried different tactics, encouraging me to lead with my upper body and "allow your legs to follow" or "feel the weight of your whole body shift from one foot to the other as you take your steps." I am not sure which of these cues clicked for me, but he noticed a sudden change.

"That was you moving in your own energy! In all these months, this is the first time I've felt it. Just like that, you switched on," Charles exclaimed. He continued to expound on being grounded in your moving body by illustrating how a dance couple "breathes"—feeling the strength of their own energy as they glide in sync, then narrowing the space between them on the intense inhale, and billowing apart on the softer exhale. This connection is crucial for the masterpiece of the whole, he explained. It was making more sense to me on a cerebral level. Now if I could just let go of my thoughts about the process and continue to allow my body to lead the way, I would be on the right track.

Later that day, I found myself caught in the web of my child's emotional turmoil despite my best efforts to be the role model of patience. My kids were pleading for my help to merge some sort of gaming membership between their Nintendo accounts. I offered an overtly frustrated and discombobulated explanation of our current technology fiasco to the customer service representative who did not follow. I lost my shit and then apologized, lost my shit and apologized, like a series of waves hitting their crescendo and then breaking peacefully on the sandy beach. I cried out to him that I couldn't believe I was putting myself through this much agony to fix something I threatened weekly to remove from my children's lives. I complained that companies like his were ruining our youth by tethering them to their screens and keeping them from experiencing the immense benefits of the wild outdoors. He said he understood. I wasn't sure if he was trying to keep my emotional wave contained or if he perhaps had kids of his own and felt a shared bond. I went with the bond. It made me feel a little better about yelling at him.

I had allowed myself to get caught up in my son's infuriated frustration. His anger became my anger. An inhale of frustration, anger, or rage was followed by an exhale of relief, apology, or forgiveness. The dance continued to repeat until the ordeal was resolved.

We are all perfect in our imperfections. We get mad, frustrated, lose our tempers, scream, cry. I had learned that chaos is more manageable, though, if we remain mindful of our own energy as we engage in our unique dances—interconnected in understanding and compassion but grounded in our own energetic flow.

Aware of some lingering tension in my body, I chose to spend the evening alone in my room. This separation from my family was not some sort of punishment for me or them. It was simply my means of self-care, and I was discovering that if I wanted to remain on the path to healing, I needed to love the parts of myself that I would have otherwise pushed down and tightly guarded after an event like that. I needed to exhale.

An hour or so later a handmade thank you card was slipped under my door:

"Thank you, Mom. We just wanted to thank you for all your help with the online membership, so we made you this card. We know that it gave you a lot of stress. Even with the anger and stress building up you stayed calm and collected on the phone and you did that for me. So thank you for that. Not only that, though, you were the one to keep me calm."

I felt a familiar pang of guilt that often followed one of my angry episodes. Even though I was learning how to let go of the mommy guilt when I wasn't my best, I realized self-forgiveness is a lifelong practice. I had been at it for years at that point. Maybe I was learning. Perhaps my outer appearance wasn't quite as disheveled as my inner world indicated. I reminded myself that awareness is an important step, and I had been self-aware throughout this ordeal. It's a marathon, not a sprint, and I was doing just fine.

CHAPTER 17

Good or Bad, Hard to Say

AS 2019 PROGRESSED INTO 2020, I CONTINUED ALONG the path of exploring my inner child and began to look at some of the emotions hidden there. At the most basic level, I often felt abandoned and alone as a child. I coped by learning to fend for myself, to cultivate and unleash my inner leopardess, to be big and fierce to mask any inkling of feeling small. Creating a strong barrier around my heart allowed me to survive without risking heartbreak. It kept me safe. Fortunately, I was graced with a nurturing mother who did the best she knew how for us. But, despite her maternal care, certain circumstances left me feeling unsafe and unloved anyway. I was cared for lovingly by my mother. I was also mothered by life circumstances that taught me you must cultivate a hard shell to survive in this world.

Although I was not a victim of abuse or crime or neglect, the little girl inside of me, my inner child, did suffer her own traumas. We all do. Childhood trauma does not have to mean that you stood witness to the murder of a parent or suffered under the hands of violence. Those deeply disturbing experiences unquestionably wound. Trauma, though, can also occur when you suddenly find yourself standing in the middle of an overwhelming grocery store without a caregiver by your side at age five. Or you walk downstairs after lights out to find your parents fighting and immediately assume that you must be to blame for their inability to work it out. These frightening but seemingly small incidents can take up ample real estate in the psyche of a child. I learned their seeds can eventually sprout into fear if not addressed properly. Fortunately for us, the growing body of neuroplasticity science definitively concludes that our brains can be rewired throughout life. With proper treatment, these detrimental neural pathways created in the wake of childhood traumas can be repaired.

This hazardous inner world was mostly outside of my awareness as I proceeded into adulthood. Until I knew it existed, I had no way of understanding how to mend it. I now know that this is what my mystery illness did for me. As you have read, it certainly wasn't an easy and obvious straight path, but after years of winding my way through this method and that modality during my healing course, I eventually surrendered to the inner recesses of my deeply guarded emotions. In facing my fears and unlocking the many safeguards I had constructed, I finally opened the fortress that protected my heart.

Without the crushing blow of a health crisis, I might never have found a way to love myself as I do now. I have come to realize that our inner worlds are much more intricate than we know; the seeds of our youth having sprouted into elaborate plants with unending branches of fear and thorns of shame. Without realizing it, we repeatedly punish ourselves for our pasts. We learn to treat ourselves the way we were treated as children. We learn to mother ourselves as we have been mothered by life.

Perhaps this is how I had learned to use my illness identity. It went beyond the comfort I once felt from many of my dis-ease symptoms—like my fatigue that held me back from committing to plans or my weak immune system that told me I was more sensitive to toxins than everyone else. Illness identity also served as a badge of disability that provided me something more enticing than the freedom from the illness itself.

The attention I desperately craved as a child that manifested in dramatic anger and attention-grabbing performances was finally received from the healthcare practitioners who treated me and the family members who came to my rescue. Once I had accrued a team of caring participants in my life after years of feeling like I was in this world alone, I had a hard time letting go of the persona that brought them to me. The cycle would continue—physical symptoms and emotional suffering which spawned the attention and care I craved—until I recognized that I preferred freedom to the childhood longing for love. Once I admitted to myself that I was truly ready to heal by letting go of the attention from others I had once longed for, the deep emotional work came more easily.

When my anger, grief, sadness (or any number of other painful emotions) went unexpressed, my body suffered.

Dis-ease was then and is now my wake-up call that inner work must take place to heal and thrive. I now know I can either accept the challenge and begin to extinguish the flames or continue to turn off, unplug, and smash the alarm bells.

Feeling the truth of my emotions—the fears hidden behind the shield of my inner leopardess—is the best tool I have learned to better understand my anger and surrender to a divinity that is wiser and more loving than I know how to be with myself. I continue to put this lesson into practice, as evidenced by a recent visit with my favorite integrative practitioner. A physician assistant, Dr. Lori Nikolic continues to find ways to work within the confines of our traditional Western medical model to reach patients who want and need so much more. She has much of the flexibility of an MD (patient oversight, prescribing privileges) but also has a PhD in naturopathic medicine and blends the two together seamlessly. *And* she accepts health insurance. After almost a decade of out-of-pocket healthcare costs in the tens, if not hundreds, of thousands of dollars, I find myself grateful for her service to the community as well as for our friendship.

As the elevator door opened and I made my way into her office, ideas ran through my head of all the things I wanted to discuss with her in my twenty or so minutes of dedicated time. I was also there for basic blood work, curious to see if my lab reports reflected how healthy I felt inside.

The receptionist greeted me with a cheerful welcome and the standard clipboard of required forms to sign. Instead of the heartfelt hello I was anticipating from

Dr. Lori, I watched in confusion as she reprimanded the new staff members and me for my late arrival.

"Haven't we discussed that patients need to be told to arrive ten minutes *before* their scheduled appointment time?" she scowled. No acknowledgment that I was standing there. No indication that I was any different than the next guy. My childhood need to be seen had just been triggered.

What? My big open smile began to close—my heart along with it. In what felt like slow motion I noticed my inner leopardess begin to forge her way to the surface. A barrage of responses formed on the tip of my tongue: *But I'm early* and *I was never told to get here ten minutes before the appointment!* And *It's not like I'm a new patient or anything. You know me!* And my son's favorite refrain, *I didn't do anything wrong!*

But instead, inner guidance stepped in, overcame the lifelong programming of my fierce leopardess, and forced me into a deep breath. This breath was key, as it gave me the moment I needed to check in with my physical body, which was visibly trembling.

Is this a tremble of anger or something else? I asked myself. And it took less than a moment more to see it for what it really was: sadness and rejection.

I took my clipboard, stepped away from the desk, and made my way to a seat in the waiting room. There, I allowed the stuffed tears to flow. In an attempt to appear as though I was simply filling out forms—head down, pen in hand—I quietly sobbed. For five minutes, I cried like a scolded child. I allowed myself to feel the shame, the rejection, the loneliness. I didn't try to analyze it or judge it. I just let the sadness breathe within me until my trembling settled, and my body felt light again.

I was called back a few minutes later, and we had a lovely albeit somewhat awkward conversation. I shared with her the emotional healing work I had been doing and she seemed genuinely moved by how it was changing me. I could also sense that she, like most people, wasn't ready to engage in this embarrassing level of self-healing anytime soon. If I were to continue doing this inner work myself, though, I needed to allow full expression of emotions no matter how inconvenient they could be. Maybe my connection to Dr. Lori would be made stronger for it.

I have felt both the chastised feeling and the unexpected rejection many times before. If I were to guess, I would say that my subconscious was catapulted right back to the wounded child inside of me. The little girl who wanted so desperately to be seen and heard. Who tried to do right. Who longed for connection. That little girl needed space to breathe. Her sadness needed room to flow. And that inconvenient place and time happened to be just the moment for the dam to break.

I find that if I can let go of my conditioned, black and white (good or bad) views about whether any given circumstance is positive or negative, then it's easier to find a sort of observer's detachment of my felt emotions as well. This is not to be confused with becoming detached from my emotions—distancing myself from them—but, instead, allowing their full expression without becoming so immersed in their weight that they pull me down into an abyss.

I stumbled across a parable that helped me accept the often uncomfortable, yet natural unfolding of life. It is the story of a Chinese farmer whose horse escaped into the hills one day. His neighbors gathered around in sympathy over his bad luck. The farmer replied, "Good or bad, hard to say." A few days later, the stallion returned with a herd of wild horses. The neighbors gathered around, congratulating him on his good fortune. "Good or bad, hard to say," said the farmer. A week later, while trying to tame one of the horses, the farmer's son was thrown from the horse and broke his leg. His neighbors thought this was very bad luck. "Good or bad, hard to say," said the farmer. Some weeks later, the Chinese army marched into the village, looking for all fit and healthy youth to join the army in battle. When the soldiers came to the farmer's house and noticed the boy's broken leg, they left him alone and continued on. While the neighbors found this to be a stroke of good luck, the farmer was not so sure. Good or bad, hard to say.

My circumstances have all the meaning I bestow upon them. The computer glitch that won't let me finish that project for the meeting tomorrow: Inconvenient. Frustrating. Anger-inducing. An opportunity to step away from my desk to take a walk: A reprieve. An excuse to delegate the task and move on.

Good or bad, hard to say.

Sometimes the moments that knock the wind out of me and bring me to my knees—the scenarios I view as very bad luck—are the very ones that bless me with gifts I could never have imagined in the days, months, or years to come. Ask someone who has raised a special needs child or has been challenged by a life-threatening illness and has come to realize the miraculous beauty in their difficult experience. Good or bad, hard to say. How can I reduce something as complex and messy and beautiful and sticky as life to good or bad? The human experience is so much richer than that.

CHAPTER 18

Inviting My Teachers

AT THIS POINT IN MY JOURNEY, IN 2021, I AM DIS-
covering that I'm here to enjoy life to the fullest.

My deepest desire is to feel whole, and my body can be
my guide if I surrender and allow it to lead the way. Listening to my fears, my difficult emotions, the whispers of
my body . . . these aren't always easy tasks.

But these signals from my body are my teachers. I can
witness these continuously changing signs, become curious, and not be shackled by them anymore. When I do
that, they move quietly and gently through me, leaving me
with just the right amount of insight. These signals ask for
my full attention—often demand it—so they can show me
the way home. Home to the fullest expression of myself.
When I find that sacred space, I see the wholeness waiting
there patiently for my return.

I have had many other teachers on this journey. One of
them, a speaking coach I worked with to help me find my
voice on stage again, listened with compassion as I told her

the story of my healing journey. Her eyes lit up, and she recited from memory a poem from 13th century Persian mystic, Rumi. His words speak beautifully about the way life happens over and over again in our quest for wholeness.

The Guest House

This being human is a guest house,
Every morning a new arrival.

A joy, a depression, a meanness,
some momentary awareness comes
as an unexpected visitor.

Welcome and entertain them all!
Even if they are a crowd of sorrows,
who violently sweep your house
empty of its furniture,
still, treat each guest honorably.
He may be clearing you out
for some new delight.

The dark thought, the shame, the malice,
meet them at the door laughing,
and invite them in.

Be grateful for whoever comes,
because each has been sent
as a guide from beyond.

AFTERWORD

I'VE CARRIED MY MEDICINE BAG, WHICH I LIKE TO imagine is adorned with fabric of ocean blues, elegant gold, and soft ivory, for my entire life. It started as a change purse with a few Flinstones vitamins and a daily dose of boiled greens; broccoli, peas, and green beans were my childhood staples. It was transferred from my hand to my shoulder as the bag expanded and became filled with prescription medications, a few surgeries, and a plethora of dietary regimens. I now have to hoist it onto my back, but it feels more balancing than burdensome. I have picked up my share of knowledge and experience, tossing out some and carefully creating interior zipped pouches to safeguard others. But one thing is certain: the majority of my bag is now comprised of items that bring me joy when I untie the string and reach inside for them.

Putting my jumbled thoughts to paper, moving my body and feeling it thank me, laughing out loud with my kids, sinking into the deliciousness of an afternoon nap, connecting with friends and loved ones in meaningful ways, exploring all that Mother Earth has to offer—activities that bring me pleasure and allow for full expression of emotions—these items are better medicine than anything I can find in a bottle. These are the remedies that not only keep me healthy, but also allow me to live fully.

RESOURCES AND FURTHER READING

CARRIE'S RESOURCES

Online Neuroplasticity Program
www.avocadotozen.com/free-your-mind-online

Clean Water Guide
www.avocadotozen.com/clean-water-guide

Mindful Eating Guide
www.avocadotozen.com/mindful-eating

Mold Illness Recovery Series
www.avocadotozen.com/from-mold-illness-to-mindfully-healed

Body Scan Meditations
www.avocadotozen.com/meditations

SUGGESTED FURTHER READING

Beck, Martha. 2001. *Finding Your Own North Star: Claiming the Life You Were Meant to Live.* New York: Three Rivers Press.
Dispenza, Joe. 2012. *Breaking the Habit of Being Yourself: How to Lose Your Mind and Create a New One.* Carlsbad, CA: Hay House.

Doidge, Norman. 2007. *The Brain That Changes Itself: Stories of Personal Triumph from the Frontiers of Brain Science*. New York: Penguin Books.

Hopper, Annie. 2014. *Wired for Healing: Remapping the Brain to Recover from Chronic and Mysterious Illnesses*. Victoria, BC: The Dynamic Neural Retraining System.

Jacobs, Gregg D. 2009. *Say Good Night to Insomnia: The Six-Week, Drug-Free Program Developed at Harvard Medical School*. New York: Henry Holt & Company, Inc.

Katie, Byron, with Stephen Mitchell. 2002. *Loving What Is: Four Questions That Can Change Your Life*. New York: Three Rivers Press.

Li, Cynthia. 2019. *Brave New Medicine: A Doctor's Unconventional Path to Healing Her Autoimmune Illness*. Oakland, CA: New Harbinger Publications.

Pollan, Michael. 2019. *How to Change Your Mind: What the New Science of Psychedelics Teaches Us About Consciousness, Dying, Addiction, Depression, and Transcendence*. New York: Penguin Books.

Sarno, John E. 1998. *The Mindbody Prescription: Healing the Body, Healing the Pain*. New York: Hachette Book Group.

Sapolsky, Robert M. 2004. *Why Zebras Don't Get Ulcers*. New York: Holt Paperbacks.

ACKNOWLEDGMENTS

I HAVE SO MUCH GRATITUDE FOR THOSE WHO LOVED and supported me while I lived and then wrote this story.

To my Jacksonville primary care physician Dr. Arpitha Ketty who, early in my journey, believed what I was going through even if she didn't have all the answers. To Dr. Aylin Ozdemir for your loving treatment of my children and your confirmation that my health challenges weren't all in my head. For those practitioners who couldn't help me and didn't have answers, I am grateful for the role you played in pushing me to do my own work of discovery.

To the practitioners who personally helped me understand the crucial role a strong gut plays in the overall health of my body, Sharon Brown, NTP, and Cynthia Li, MD. Dr. Li, thank you also for your courage to speak up so boldly in the mainstream medical community.

To my original soul tribe—Kintu Patel, Ragda Deeb, Chez Leeby, Kim Purcell, and Martha Cesery. Your friendships came into my life at the perfect moment and introduced me to the spiritual path that ultimately allowed me to heal as fully as I have.

To all the friends I leaned on along the way including, but not limited to, Heather Tesch, Kay Hutcheson, Linda Gingerich, Monica Velez, Heather Marineau, Laura Bushey-Garwood, and Kathryn Gordon. And to Karen Odierna for creating such an amazing space in Sarasota in which to treat myself to the cleanest juice on the planet while always getting to chat about the latest health-related topics with fun, like-minded people.

To my holistic healing team and the lightworkers who opened my eyes to so many incredible modalities, Don, Claire, Marci, Frannie, Desiree, Kristi, Melinda, Jason, Lori, Belinda, and Edwin.

To our fantastic mold remediation experts—Jenny Canning, Luis Mahiquez, and Will Spates. Will, your dedication and passion to indoor air quality protocols will be your legacy. May you rest in peace.

To my fellow Wayfinder coaches—Julie Edge, Shannon Gilcrease, and Diane Douiyssi. Your countless hours of coaching and loving friendships provided me with such beautiful support as I turned the corner and ascended in my healing journey.

To Gail Larsen, whose Transformational Speaking course helped me birth this transformational manuscript. To all those who read and edited the various stages of the book—Susan Kilman, Kara Bumgarner, Janice Harper, Allison Serrell, Maggie Langrick and the incredible team at Wonderwell. To my dear friend, Ellen Brown—having you be a part of the development of this book has brought me immense joy. Reconnecting with you has been my honor and privilege. Thank you.

To Curtis, J, and Jordan, for your openness to learning about my journey and the work I do now. Being the oldest sibling keeps me on my toes so that I can hopefully impart some health and wellness wisdom on to you.

To my parents who, though only mentioned in limited strands weaved into this memoir, decorated me with innumerable gifts. Mom, thank you for exemplifying the beauty of a self-starting, entrepreneurial woman. Dad, thank you for showing me that it's more than okay to question the norms and think for myself. I love that our relationship today is closer than ever.

And most of all, to my family, Matt, Colin, and Bennett—my heart, my happiness, and my reason for thriving on this journey. If my experience can help you lead healthier, heart-centered lives then it will have been worth every bump and bruise I endured along the way.

INDEX

ABOUT THE AUTHOR

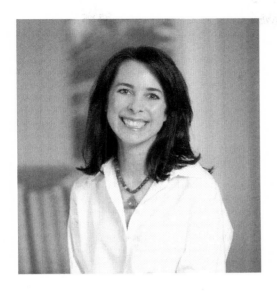

CARRIE ECKERT is a mind-body health coach and "mystery illness" mentor. In addition to experiencing her own healing journey, she holds a Master's degree in Health and Wellness Coaching. Carrie has trained with and learned from industry-leading professionals including Martha Beck, Annie Hopper, Byron Katie, and Dr. Joe Dispenza. Carrie now uses neuroplasticity techniques and embodiment practices to help those challenged with physical and emotional dis-ease to heal. She lives in Sarasota, Florida with her husband, two sons, and her Brittany spaniel. Visit her at www.AvocadoToZen.com.

Made in the USA
Coppell, TX
06 May 2021

55168937R10134